THE ART & SCIENCE OF
UNDERMINING
CANCER

THE **ART & SCIENCE** OF
UNDERMINING
CANCER

STRATEGIES TO
SLOW·CONTROL·REVERSE

FRANCISCO CONTRERAS, MD
DANIEL E. KENNEDY, MC

The Art & Science of Undermining Cancer

Book Cover Design by Marcela Contreras-Santini & Daniel E. Kennedy

Formatting by Daniel E. Kennedy

Illustrations and graphic design by Marcela Contreras-Santini

Additional graphic design by Ana Karehn Nieva

Watercolor painting of Dr. Ernesto Contreras, Sr. by Medez Calvillo

Photography by Dwight Vallely & Ana Karehn Nieva

ISBN: 978-1-953552-00-6
Paperback ISBN: 978-1-953552-99-0
eBook ISBN: 978-1-953552-01-3

First Edition: September 2020

DEDICATION

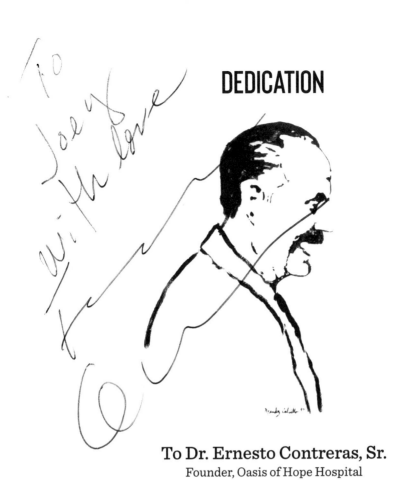

To Dr. Ernesto Contreras, Sr.
Founder, Oasis of Hope Hospital

You were a pioneer of holistic care and alternative cancer treatments. Your compassion led the fight against cancer. Your vision, medical expertise and love healed tens of thousands of people worldwide. Your healing legacy lives in our hearts and blesses our patients who receive total care for their bodies, minds and spirits.

WHAT EXPERTS SAY

Ralph W. Moss, PhD

In 1976, while I was still working for Memorial Sloan-Kettering Cancer Center in New York, I snuck away from a scientific meeting in California to visit to Oasis of Hope Hospital in Tijuana. There I met with its founder, Ernesto Contreras, MD. Although Dr. Contreras was sometimes pilloried in the US media as a "cancer quack" exploiting desperate patients, the man I met was clearly a humane and caring individual, who was doing his best to improve the health of mostly very ill cancer patients. In our meeting, he made no exaggerated claims for his treatment. Most of his patients were either given no hope or were offered treatments that seemed to them worse than the disease. Since that time, cancer treatment has improved in many ways and is more humane than the typical treatment of the 1970s. Yet, there is still a crying need for complementary and alternative clinics, such as Oasis of Hope, that offer treatments not generally available at standard hospitals. I wish them well in offering all scientifically valid treatments that are in the interest of cancer patients worldwide.

—Ralph W. Moss, PhD
Researcher, Author and
Founder of Moss Reports
www.mossreports.com

Satya Prakash, PhD

This book is a must-read for physicians, cancer caregivers and families who would like to understand the complexities of cancer and available total-cancer-care resources for healing. The book details the most updated science about cancer and provides essential scientific tools for total cancer care, specifically managing and undermining cancer with much needed human touch. The book is a lucid reading full of modern knowledge, tools and a comprehensive collection of protocols developed over sixty years. It presents the work from the globally known cancer therapy and healing experience of Oasis of Hope.

—Satya Prakash, PhD
Professor of Biomedical Engineering,
Experimental Medicine, Physiology,
Artificial Cell and Organs & Experimental Surgery
McGill University

Frank Cousineau

The Contreras name and Alternative/Integrative Therapies have been synonymous since 1963. This latest book from the progeny of Dr. Ernesto Contreras, Sr., artfully blends the history of a prominent family and a movement. It also provides a comprehensive and easy to understand compendium of cancer treatments that integrate the growing number of alternative cancer protocols combined with the judicious use of of conventional modalities, along with inspiring histories of successfully treated patients. Dr. Contreras describes how each element of the patient treatment program is chosen, and more importantly for the patient, why. In *The Art & Science of Undermining Cancer*, you will learn the Oasis of Hope approach to cancer as it:

- Addresses the strengths of cancer, as a disease, and leverages the weaknesses of cancer.
- Explores opportunities to control cancer, and mitigates the threat of cancer recurrence.

The Oasis of Hope approach is patient-centric and provides care for the whole person—body, mind and spirit. Having personally experienced much of the Oasis of Hope history, I strongly recommend The Art & Science of Undermining Cancer. It will provide help and hope for your body, understanding for your mind and added fortitude for your spirit.

—Frank Cousineau
President, Cancer Control Society
www.CancerControlSociety.com

Sophie Sabbage

When I was diagnosed with terminal lung cancer in 2014, and my only medical option was palliative whole-brain radiation, I approached several clinics around the world. Dr. Contreras was the only one to take me in, to give me hope. He is not just a pioneer of integrated oncology. He also treated me with faith. Imagine a doctor who merges chemotherapy with green juice, radiotherapy with hyperthermia, surgery with laughter, and science with faith! Since then, I have walked with acceptance, knowledge, medicine and power. I'm not cured. I've had multiple brain tumours four times, including leptomeningeal disease, but I'm yet to have whole-brain radiotherapy. I've nearly died twice, but I'm tumour free as I write. I've far outrun my use-by date because I have a raft of options that were not offered to me when I could hardly breathe from the tumour in my lung, and wishing for something different. I have Dr. Contreras to thank for a big chunk of that. This book is needed. Read it.

—Sophie Sabbage
Sunday Times bestselling author of
The Cancer Whisperer
www.SophieSabbage.com

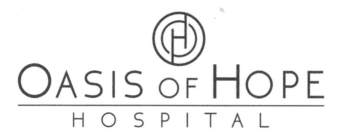

OUR MISSION

Oasis of Hope is

Caring
for the whole person–body, mind and spirit,
Sharing
the healing power of faith, hope and love, and
Advancing
medical science to end cancer,
one person at a time.

CARING • SHARING • ADVANCING

CONTENTS

PREFACE

President Richard Nixon declared war on cancer on December 23, 1971, when he signed the National Cancer Act that gave autonomy to the National Cancer Institute and increased research funding by $700 million over the first seven years. It was believed that a cure would be found within ten years. Nearly fifty years later, we are no closer to the cure. In absolute numbers, the harsh reality is that twice as many people will be diagnosed with cancer, and twice as many people will die from cancer in 2021 than in 1971.

Though the probability of surviving cancer is higher now than five decades ago, it isn't because of advances in treatment. More people survive cancer now because of improvements in screening, education and lifestyle changes. Early detection and diagnosis allow cancer to be found and treated in the early stages. Cure rates are excellent in the early stages for many types of cancers, because most people do not die from a primary tumor. Metastases are deadly, making it very challenging to recover from stage four cancers.

This book has been written because chemotherapy, radiation and surgery are failing patients with advanced-stage metastatic cancer. Not only are they failing significantly, but they also have intolerable side effects, and they devastate a patient's quality of life. The new wave of targeted therapies and treatments that are emerging from genome sequencing are promising, but they are also cost-prohibitive and still under development.

Cutting edge technologies, such as the CRISPR genome editing tool, have mesmerized those working in the oncology field. They have us daydreaming of how we will one day put an end to cancer with gene and cell-based therapies. Whether it is pie in the sky thinking or not, DNA modifying cancer treatment is far from available to patients. People need alternatives to traditional cancer therapy now.

The Art & Science of Undermining Cancer has been written to share a revolutionary approach to cancer treatment—one that is holistic and leverages research-based alternative therapies and employs traditional oncology drugs in non-traditional ways. The book is written in two parts.

Part One gives the back story of how Oasis of Hope Hospital came to be, and how its multi-pronged holistic cancer treatment protocols were developed and advanced over the last fifty-seven years. It also gives an overview of how cancer first develops, how it progresses and why alternatives are needed.

Part Two explains how Oasis of Hope treatment strategies work synergistically to undermine cancer. The chapters parallel *The Art of War*, the compilation of the war tactics developed and employed by the great General Sun Tzu in ancient China. By the way, you will see some Chinese characters on many of the pages in this book. Those characters symbolize the words *Art*, *Science*, *Undermine* and *Cancer*. It is just a tip of the hat to one of the most brilliant strategists in history. The reference to war tactics is relevant to anyone facing advanced-stage cancer because they are fighting for their lives with all of their might.

If you need to find answers quickly, feel free to jump forward to **Part Two**. If you have time to read **Part One**, please do. Knowing the back story, and how cancer works, could make the book more meaningful. Hopefully, you will enjoy getting to know my grandfather, and founder of Oasis of Hope Hospital, Dr. Ernesto Contreras, Sr., as you read through the first chapter.

If you, or your loved one, is facing cancer, and doctors are not providing treatment options that make sense, this book may help motivate you to keep fighting the good fight, and provide practical and research-based ways to go about it.

—Daniel E. Kennedy, MC

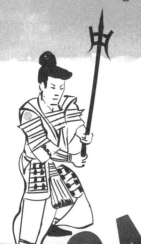
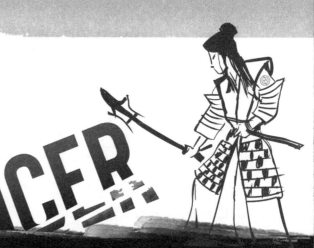

THE ART AND SCIENCE OF UNDERMINING

艺术 科学 削弱 癌

CANCER

PART ONE

ONE

TOTAL CARE APPROACH

Caring for the whole person—body, mind and spirit.

I n a pueblo outside Guadalajara, Mexico, a young mother made her way through a crowded dirt street carrying her two-year-old back home from the market. She wanted to get close to the town's mayor to hear if an attack was about to happen. Unfortunately, the confusion and the noisy crowd made it hard to see further than five feet in front of where she was standing. The restless little boy wiggled out of her arms and slipped away between people. She panicked until she saw her son with his arms wrapped around her husband's leg. The mayor raised his voice, and an eerie quiet came over the crowd. He shared a report of violent clashes between the Mexican Army and the rebel militia. It was evident that the rebel forces' path of retreat was leading directly to the pueblo. Hearing such terrifying news was a heartbreaking moment for the young mother and the townspeople. The two-year-old boy tugged on his father's pant leg. His father looked down and reassuringly said, "No te preocupes Ernesto, everything will be alright."

Manuel Contreras was the general manager of the town's flour mill. He was confident that with his influence and resources, he would be able to protect his son, wife, and four other children. However, as the future would reveal, he would be unable to overcome the terrible loss they were about to experience as a family—as a people.

That day, the Contreras family went from living in the most exquisite house in the pueblo to being completely homeless. This real-life *From Prada To Nada* story left the family destitute. Millions of people across Mexico lost everything during the Mexican Revolution. Overnight, the Contreras had become war refugees who were desperately trying to survive and keep the family together. Little Ernesto did not know what to think and do with the intense life lessons he was learning at such a tender age. This struggle against overwhelming opposition stole away his innocence and lit a fire in his heart to fight for the ones he loved and care for all who were suffering.

POLITICS HAD BECOME SELF-SERVING

The Mexican Revolution, which started in 1910 under the leadership of Francisco Madero, provoked many negative side effects. The Contreras family was part of the collateral damage of war. For the previous thirty years, Mexico had been under the dictatorship of Porfirio Díaz, whose corrupt rule favored the elite and exploited the poor. Initially, Madero's efforts were unsuccessful, and he had to seek refuge on the northern side of the border in Texas. After doing so, he gained support from Texas and worked hard to develop strategies to rekindle the revolutionary fire.

By 1911, the Mexican Revolution was blazing with Madero at the helm. He was supported initially by Pancho Villa, who led the charge in the north, and Emiliano Zapata, who commanded the rebels in the south. There were countless stories of Mexican civilians caught amidst battles trying to survive, and many of them went unnoticed. The rebel forces promised hope but often commandeered resources and belongings from innocent people to advance their cause.

The rebels opposed how the political system and government had become self-serving. The politicians were not acting in the interests of the people. It would take a revolution to change the system.

MEDICINE HAD BECOME SELF-SERVING

In the same years of the Mexican Revolution, medicine was going through a radical transformation from a healing art to a medical science. Gone would be the days where the doctor was a cherished member of every family in town. That warm, healing relationship would give way to cold, calculating clinical technicians. Medical office consultations would replace house calls, laboratory tests would substitute intuition, and diagnostic competencies would supplant caring and compassion.

While drug therapy, medical devices and diagnostic tools improved, medical schools indoctrinated their students to be scientists and technicians who would look at the data without compromising objectivity by interacting with patients. It was frowned upon to get to know a patient due to the risk of forming an emotional attachment that could distort a physician's judgment.

In the new medical science model, the ends justified the means. It didn't matter what negative side effects a patient would have to suffer as long as the goal of destroying the disease was being pursued. In some cases, patients would die from the treatment before the diseases had time to take their lives.

In the name of scientific advancement, developing drugs and medical devices became an industry, and patients became

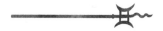

its collateral damage. Medical institutions and pharmaceutical companies had become self-serving. Many doctors were no longer acting in the interests of their patients. It would take a revolution to change the system.

A MEDICAL REVOLUTIONARY

Here we present the story of that two-year-old boy named Ernesto Contreras, who survived the Mexican Revolution and grew up to start a medical revolution. The inciting incident causing the Contreras family to flee to Mexico City happened when the rebels seized their house and left them out on the street. Once in Mexico's capital, Ernesto's mother found work as a teacher in a government school. His father went further north looking for work but was unsuccessful and never returned to the family. He left his wife alone to fend for their five children.

Imagine the wages of a government-employed teacher in Mexico City during the 1930s. There was never enough money to go around, but somehow the family survived, and Ernesto became a young man full of hope, dreams and determination. His uncle recognized Ernesto's potential and paid an unexpected visit to their home with some surprising news. He had taken it upon himself to sign Ernesto up for the admittance test to the Mexican Army School. Considering his terrible childhood memories of soldiers, Ernesto had no interest in becoming a military man. At the same time, he saw it as an opportunity to make some money to help support his mother and siblings. He deeply desired to see his family go to bed with full stomachs instead of empty bellies. He took the test and was accepted. Though he received a pittance for pay, he gave all of the pesos he earned to his mother, and it helped. His real payoff was learning medicine and graduating as a doctor and surgeon from the prestigious Army Medical School, which continues to be the top medical school in Mexico.

Though he had never wanted to become a warrior, his circumstances led him into the military field. He quickly discovered that while foot soldiers trained to fight and take away the lives of the enemy, military doctors trained to fight to preserve the lives of their Army brothers and sisters. He found his passion for saving lives through this experience. The Army taught him discipline. One of Ernesto's good qualities that helped him progress in the Army was his methodic nature. It was his way of thinking and turning his thoughts into actions, that made him an ideal fit for the Army. Little did he know that later in life, he would use military strategies as an integral part of his approach to cancer treatment.

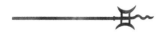

Ernesto's ferocious appetite for learning transformed him into an excellent doctor who was an expert in his field. His decision to join the Army, and go the military medical school, was a significant turning point in his life. Things got a lot better for him.

At the time of his graduation from medical school in 1939, no one could have predicted that he would become a medical revolutionary. That time would come, but first, he would serve some of the most impoverished populations in Mexico. He wouldn't do it alone.

LOVE WAS IN THE AIR

Ernesto must have looked quite handsome in his military officer's uniform because he successfully wooed and persuaded the beautiful Rita Pulido to marry him. She was a woman of strong character and great conviction. Rita informed Ernesto that her commitment to the Lord Jesus Christ was paramount. She would only marry a good Christian man. Ernesto did not think twice when she invited him to know Jesus as his Lord and Savior. He embraced Christianity with all his heart, and they were married on May 26, 1941. Ernesto experienced the great love and compassion of Christ and this helped him develop a deeper devotion to his profession and his patients.

MOLDING A BRILLIANT MEDICAL MIND

With Rita at his side, Ernesto accepted his appointment to serve the healthcare needs of people living in the small town of San Luis Potosi, Mexico. There were no medical facilities, running water or electricity. In extreme cases, he had no other option than to perform life-saving surgeries on his kitchen table while simultaneously training Rita to be a surgical assistant and anesthesiologist. It was in that town where their first child, Estela del Carmen, was born in 1942. Once he completed his two-year social service requirement, the Army surprised him by sending him to Boston, Massachusetts, to advance his medical knowledge and diagnostic skills.

A HARVARD MEDICAL SCHOOL FELLOW

Dr. Ernesto Contreras, Sr. had specialized in pathology and oncology in Mexico and was blessed to further train in pediatric pathology at Harvard Medical School's Boston Children's Hospital. He excelled and thoroughly enjoyed becoming a master diagnostician, but he felt that something was missing. He wouldn't find what he was looking for until 1960—twenty-one years after he had graduated from medical school.

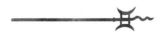

THE TOTAL CARE APPROACH'S INSPIRATION

Ernesto appreciated all of the advances in medical knowledge and technology, but he took issue with the treatment philosophy that detached the physician from the patient. The professors at medical school taught that the scientific method was the new and effective way to practice medicine. Remember, he was in medical school at the time that healthcare was evolving and becoming an industry. It's when health insurance was birthed and quickly changed from protecting a patient to a profit-making machine. Blue Cross made its offering of health insurance right after the great stock market crash of 1929. By 1939, the year Ernesto graduated from medical school, more than three million people had subscribed and were paying insurance premiums, which fueled the new medical machine.[1] Doctors were the essential part of growing the industry that today represents twenty percent of the gross national product in the United States.

Medical professors taught Ernesto to observe, take notes, utilize diagnostic tests, evaluate and treat. Engagement with patients was avoided to minimize the loss of objectivity. When conducting rounds, doctors were encouraged not to use the patients' names. Instead, the patients were referred to by their diagnosis. They would observe the kidney stone in room 214, the lung carcinoma in 510 and the fractured femur in 102. This impersonal medical method went against his beliefs.

The business of medicine created dissonance in his soul. Throughout the first twenty years of his career, he was dismayed with the treatment of patients. He believed the impersonal approach in hospitals was illogical, impractical and would lead to poor results. He thought there could be a better patient treatment model, but he didn't know where to find it. He surely didn't expect to find the answer to modern medicine's failure while visiting ancient Greek ruins. But that's precisely what happened.

A TRIP OF A LIFETIME

Ernesto and Rita had a total of six children. Their daughter Estela had grown up and married a young pastor. In 1960, Ernesto and Rita invited Estela, and her husband David, on a trip around the globe. It was inspiring and life-changing for Ernesto. The tour took them to see the wonders of the world, including The Great Wall of China and the Egyptian Pyramids. When they went to Turkey, they had a free day. The tour guide, knowing that Ernesto was a medical doctor, suggested they visit the ancient Greek healing center of the demi-god Asclepius in Pergamum. It was there he had an epiphany.

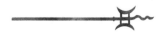

The Asclepion healing center had three main sections. The patients would receive emotional therapies for the healing of their minds and souls first. They would walk through a tunnel that had small openings in the walls. Healers on the outside would speak through the openings making positive statements such as, "You are going to be fine," "You are going to make it," and "You are going to heal." The patients would also receive spiritual counseling and treatments for their bodies.

The modernization of medical science has distanced doctors from the art of healing.

Touring this ancient healing center sparked Ernesto's sudden understanding that modern medicine failed because it focused solely on the patients' bodies. Doctors were essentially trained to be body mechanics. But God had created humans as triune beings where our three parts—body, mind and spirit—are one. Doctors got caught up in science of medicine, and had lost the art of healing. He decided that he would be a doctor of art and science that would administer total care to his patients. He would provide physical, emotional and spiritual resources to help patients experience true and total healing.

In ancient times, Pergamum was an important location for the advancement of knowledge. It is also where scholars believe the temple of Zeus was located, and the altar was considered the seat of Satan. Ernesto was convinced that if physicians were getting results using a Greek mythology foundation, there was tremendous potential for a treatment modality founded on Jesus Christ the *Rock*, the *Great Physician*, the *Healer*. Touring the ancient healing center galvanized his beliefs. It was then he formed two guiding principles that physicians at Oasis of Hope follow to this day:

- Love your patient as yourself. — Inspired by Jesus Christ
- First, do no harm. —Hippocrates

Dr. Ernesto Contreras, Sr. had been trained as an Army medical doctor, a pathologist, an oncologist, a Harvard Medical School Fellow in pediatric pathology and an ordained minister in the Methodist church. He had developed his *total care approach* to treating patients. He didn't know what was coming next, but he was prepared and ready.

THE BIRTH OF OASIS OF HOPE

In 1955, the Mexican Army transferred Dr. Contreras, Sr. to Tijuana. He was the first pathologist and oncologist ever in

the northwest of Mexico. There were so few specialists that he crossed the border weekly to San Diego, California, where he performed tissue analysis at Mercy Hospital. A decade later, he would also work at the University of California San Diego Hospital. Relocating Dr. Contreras, Sr. to Tijuana was God's way of positioning him for an encounter that would lead to the launching of Oasis of Hope Hospital.

In 1963, a patient named Cecile Hoffman came to Ernesto with very intriguing circumstances. She was participating in a clinical trial conducted in Canada. The doctors said her condition would allow her to live just a few more months. She became too weak to travel to Canada. She looked for a doctor in San Diego that would continue to give her the injections of the medication she had brought back with her from Canada. The treatment was experimental and could not be administered in the United States. Cecil shared her dilemma with her pastor in El Cajon, California. Her pastor knew Dr. Contreras, Sr. and recommended that she visit him.

So that is how she came to Dr. Contreras, Sr. She explained her situation and showed him the laetrile (also known as amygdalin and Vitamin B17) she had brought back with her from Canada. After listening to her whole story, he felt compassion. He agreed to administer the therapy on the condition that if he saw any negative side effects, he would discontinue treatment immediately. After treating her for a week, he noticed a positive change in her general condition. She began to gain strength and put the weight back on that she had lost due to being ill with cancer. Soon, Cecil went into full remission. She became a cancer victor, and she was the first of tens of thousands of people who would travel to Oasis of Hope for alternative cancer treatment. Dr. Contreras, Sr.'s small consultation office was quickly overwhelmed by the number of patients seeking his help. His wife saw the need. She drew up plans and built a hospital for their patients. This is how Oasis of Hope got its start. It was the first hospital in Mexico to offer alternative holistic and integrative cancer treatment in North America.

Dr. Contreras, Sr.'s natural methods of treating cancer were as effective as conventional cancer treatments without the negative side effects like hair loss and severe nausea. It may be why Oasis of Hope inspired many copycats. A number of centers in Tijuana belong to doctors who were trained at our hospital before opening up their clinics. Imitation may be the sincerest form of flattery, but using part of our trademarked name to draw attention may be a little over the line.

Today, Oasis of Hope Hospital continues to lead the way in the development of innovative treatments and holistic care. It may be the only hospital in Mexico that starts off each day with a pastor leading devotions and worship songs to minister to our patients' souls.

At our humble beginnings, Dr. Contreras, Sr. was inspired by God to treat patients like family members with body, mind and spirit medicine. He intuitively knew that amygdalin was just a piece of the puzzle, and integrating conventional therapies would be beneficial. Oasis of Hope became the treatment center where the best of alternative and traditional medicine would be available to patients.

Dr. Ernesto Contreras, Sr. pioneered the integrative holistic treatment method called *The Total Care Approach*

LABELED A QUACK

The journey was not a walk in the park. Things changed for him once he started treating patients with amygdalin and other alternative therapies. Even though he was the co-founder of the associations of pathology and oncology, Dr. Contreras, Sr. was persecuted professionally by colleagues that had once exalted him. He dared to share his serendipitous experience in Pergamum and his *total care approach*. He was shocked that his colleagues rejected his concept and turned their backs on him. It was a rude awakening. Putting patients' needs before medical industry norms would become a road he traveled alone until his sons joined his practice many years later.

In the 1970s, Dr. Contreras, Sr. had already been unjustly labeled a "quack" by medical institutions. To add insult to injury, the US government accused him of supplying drugs for patients to smuggle from Mexico into the United States.[2] Imagine treating amygdalin like heroine. The case against Dr. Contreras, Sr. was ruled unconstitutional and thrown out of court. Soon after, President Ronald Reagan promoted legislation giving pharmaceutical companies in the USA the ability to export non-FDA approved drugs to be sold in foreign countries.[3] This law also gave American citizens, who sought medical care abroad, the right to bring back prescription medication from a foreign country. Through all of the opposition and difficulties Dr. Contreras, Sr. endured, he never lost sight of God. The personal attacks did not deter him. Love for his patients was more potent than threats from those protecting their interests. This medical revolution to treat the whole person opened the eyes of many people to the benefits of alternative methods of treating cancer. Dr. Ernesto Contreras, Sr. was the first doctor in Mexico to treat cancer patients with amygdalin.[4] Amygdalin was the catalyst for Dr. Contreras, Sr. to establish his hospital. Oasis of Hope is the birthplace of alternative cancer treatments in Mexico. It was also the epicenter for the most significant cancer related-controversy of the 1960s and 1970s.

Around this time, numerous scientists and legislators argued against the efficacy and safety of amygdalin. However, this debate came to an end by the late 1970s when proponents of amygdalin conclusively touted its cancer-killing properties under the strategy devised by Dr. Contreras, Sr. Yet, even then, its opponents stated that amygdalin was ineffective at best, and dangerously toxic at worst.

**Oasis of Hope is the birthplace of
alternative cancer treatment in Mexico.**

ARGUMENTS AGAINST AMYGDALIN

The first argument made against amygdalin was that it would provoke cyanide poisoning in patients. Amygdalin is a cyanogenic glucoside. Though it has a cyanide radical, no cancer patient has ever shown signs of cyanide poisoning from amygdalin in clinical studies. Opponents to amygdalin point to a case study with children who suffered cyanide poisoning after ingesting it in bitter almonds.[5]   This is a false equivalence because it is comparing healthy children eating bitter almonds with cancer patients receiving intravenous infusions of amygdalin.   Oasis of Hope has treated tens of thousands of patients over the last six decades, and not one has ever experienced any symptom of cyanide poisoning.   There is a physiological mechanism that directs amygdalin against cancer cells without harming healthy cells.

For a better understanding, look at how amygdalin works. The use of amygdalin is safe because the mitochondrial enzyme *rhodanese* detoxifies cyanide.[6] Rhodanese is abundant in healthy cells because they are aerobic. But, malignant cells are anaerobic and do not have rhodanese, which makes it much more difficult for the cyanide to biodegrade in cancer cells. This mitochondrial enzyme is why amygdalin is safe for healthy cells and detrimental to cancer cells.

LIFE EXTENSION DOESN'T PROVE EFFICACY?

The second argument against amygdalin is that it is ineffective. In the 1970s, cancer researchers at Memorial Sloan Kettering conducted studies that provided mixed results. Part

of the research included inviting Dr. Ernesto Contreras, Sr. to present case studies from Oasis of Hope. He showed X-rays of patients who had experienced cancer control and were living ten years after their diagnoses. However, the researchers rejected the case studies on the grounds that complete tumor destruction had not been achieved. **They indicated that life extension was not proof of the efficacy of a drug; whereas tumor regression was a valid measure, regardless of whether the patient lived or died.**

As an institution, Memorial Sloan Kettering concluded that amygdalin was not a viable cancer treatment, though its researchers presented cases of patients who benefited from it.[7] Its primary researcher, Dr. Kanematsu Sugiura, published his conclusion, which stated that *"...it [amygdalin] shows a strong inhibitory effect on the development of lung metastases in mice."* He observed that one hundred percent of the mice with breast cancer tumors not treated with amygdalin experienced lung metastases. In contrast, only twenty-two percent of the mice treated with amygdalin experienced metastases.

Considering Dr. Sugiura's findings, it is difficult to understand why Memorial Sloan Kettering did not proceed with clinical trials, and   dismissed amygdalin instead. Unfortunately, the National Cancer Institute accepted

Memorial Sloan Kettering's report discrediting amygdalin.[8] The NCI's position is that amygdalin has shown some limited benefits to, but no long-term results have been observed.

WHY OASIS OF HOPE USES AMYGDALIN

The NCI does not support the use of amygdalin alone, but says it's promising when used in combination with other therapies, including pancreatic enzymes and high-dose Vitamin C. We wonder if the NCI realizes that its position on amygdalin is practically an endorsement of the Oasis of Hope protocol? Thank you NCI!

We consider amygdalin to be a potent adjuvant therapy. We agree with the NCI that amygdalin is not a cure for cancer. It is not a standalone drug that can reverse the disease. But, clinical studies support the use of amygdalin as an adjuvant in patients suffering from malignancies.[9] Studies the 1970s that discredited amygdalin are quickly being supplanted by studies published from 2004 to 2019. These recent studies conclude that amygdalin possesses anticancer qualities including, *"Decomposing carcinogenic substances in the body, killing cancer cells, blocking nutrient source of tumor cells, and inhibiting cancer cell growth."*[10] The evidence is growing that supports amygdalin's chemo-preventive properties and its ability to stabilize tumors and slow growth. Studies are finding that amygdalin has attributes that were previously not known. For example, amygdalin is a potent neurotrophic agent, which suggests that it could help repair nerve damage from chemotherapy. It also has the potential to be used to treat neurodegenerative diseases.[11]

Ongoing studies demonstrate amygdalin's effect on stabilizing tumors and slowing growth.[12]   It is an active anti-inflammatory agent which also inhibits cancer's ability to progress.[13, 14]

MORE THAN 100,000 PATIENTS TREATED SINCE 1963

It is refreshing to see so many studies, published as recently as 2019, which provide the scientific evidence of the efficacy of amygdalin.   There will always be opponents.   Many of them prefer to sell expensive and ineffective chemotherapies.   The opposition rages on despite the pro scientific evidence of amygdalin. The opponents have enough power and have leaned on Google to prohibit any website using the word amygdalin to advertise. Wow! But Oasis of Hope won't dismiss amygdalin.

Oasis of Hope has administered amygdalin to more than 100,000 patients since 1963, and there has never been one case of cyanide poisoning. There are countless stories of benefits patients received from the treatment. Oasis of Hope will continue to champion amygdalin for its patients and point to the recent studies that indicate that it can be instrumental in promoting apoptosis, thus inhibiting the progression of many cancers including prostate,[15] cervical,[16] liver,[17] lung[18] and colon.[19]

The immune system is the most potent God-given anticancer fighting agent.

PROMOTION OF THE IMMUNE SYSTEM

Dr. Contreras, Sr. may have been known as the most experienced physician with the effective use of amygdalin, but equally as important was his commitment to promoting a patient's immune system. At the core of treating a patient's body is the rebuilding of the immune system—the most potent God-given anticancer fighting agent.

A HEALING LEGACY

Dr. Contreras, Sr. taught the doctors at Oasis of Hope to treat the patient, not the disease. Most oncology programs focus on tumor destruction, and the patient's quality of life is secondary if considered at all. This approach is utterly wrong, backward, upside down and inside out. Fortunately, Oasis of Hope's *total care approach* is revolutionary because of its founding principles established by Dr. Ernesto Contreras, Sr. back in the 1960s. He taught us to love our patients as we love ourselves. Therefore, we only offer treatments to a patient that we would take ourselves if faced with the same diagnosis, prognosis and disease progression. He also reminded us that doctors must not harm our patients. We only give treatments that will help the patient and will not provoke intense negative side effects that destroy the patient's quality of life. Loving patients and caring for the whole person—body, mind and spirit—are what make up the healing legacy of Dr. Ernesto Contreras, Sr.

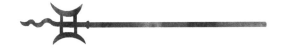

STORY OF HOPE

Rick Hill • High-grade Embryonal Cell Carcinoma, Stage 3• 1974

In 1974, I was twenty-four and at the Mayo Clinic for ten hours of cancer surgery. Post-surgery chemotherapy was mandatory, but the cancer was so widespread in my lymphatic system that the prognosis was not good.

Just before starting chemo, a letter arrived from a Baptist pastor telling me I should go to a clinic in Tijuana and take something made from apricots instead of chemo. Really? If life had an eraser, I would have used it. I told my family I was leaving Mayo, and they were furious.

Now, before you jump all over my family, what if your son, daughter, or sibling was at the Mayo Clinic in Rochester with terminal cancer and an insurance policy that would cover the full cost of treatment, but he decided to leave for a foreign country which is not known to be a medical Mecca? He wouldn't be able to use insurance and would have to depend on the generosity of family and friends to raise the money. You may feel just like my brother who said, "We always knew you were stupid; we just didn't know how stupid."

I had high-grade embryonal cell carcinoma, stage 3. When I told my surgeon at Mayo that I was leaving, he said I would not survive that decision, but cynically said, "Well, at least it's warm in Tijuana."

When I arrived at Oasis of Hope, I felt like Alice in Wonderland. Nothing was familiar. There were no health food stores where I was from. I hear speakers all the time say that unless we first believe in ourselves, we probably won't succeed—at anything. Well, I'm here to testify that sometimes you just go with your gut even when you have doubts and are scared nearly to death.

Dr. Ernesto Contreras, Sr. led with love and had a stellar medical career both in the United States and Mexico; but it was his attitude that gave me the confidence to stay and be "all in." I also owed it to the members at my church in New Ulm, Minnesota, who took up a collection to send me for treatment. I committed to holding nothing back and doing whatever they said in order to live. That was 46 years ago! What was "all in" for me? It was to follow their instructions for as long as it took. My program was simple...but not easy. Basically, I took a 3-gram injection of laetrile once a day for 21 days, and then returned home to detox and follow the plan:

1. Eat only organic food, 80% raw, which is mostly fruit and vegetables salads.
2. I ate meat just once a week, usually on Sundays after church, and even then it was organic chicken or beef, maybe 6 oz. serving—and along with beans and cornbread, I was transported back to my Southern roots. On Mondays, I'd start my juice fast—usually watermelon, and continue that until Wednesday evening. At the end of the fast, I did colonics.
3. Of course, I eliminated most sugar, processed foods, bleached flours, etc.
4. I prayed a lot in those days and decided that if I lived, I would dedicate the rest of my life to helping people get well.

If I could have ordered my cancer treatment like a deli sandwich, I would have said, "I'll have the laetrile, hold the Mayo, with a side of enzymes." This strict program was followed religiously for <u>five full years</u>, and at that point, I shifted to a more organic Mediterranean diet and allowed myself small amounts of treats. I always asked myself if the food I was eating had the needed live enzymes in it to help me use it? A Snickers candy bar never fits that definition.

I'll be seventy in November, and thank God I became ill so young because at this age, I'm about 150 pounds, no high blood pressure or cholesterol, and currently taking no prescription drugs other than some eye drops for glaucoma. When I visit the grocery store and see people my age barely able to walk and see what's in their shopping baskets, I think about their response, "Well no one lives forever and I want to enjoy life." Really? Are they enjoying life? There's good news in this book if you use it.

—Rick Hill
San Diego, California
USA

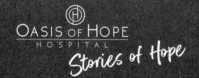

TWO

ABOUT CANCER

Cancer, above all other diseases, has countless secondary causes.
But even for cancer, there is only one prime cause: metabolism.
— Otto Warburg

Angelina Jolie made headlines in May of 2013. No, it wasn't for wearing Billy Bob Thornton's blood around her neck, her rocky relationship with Brad Pitt, nor her work as a United Nations humanitarian.[1] It was a personal choice that would be consequential to women's health. Her decisions and actions in 2013, and then again in 2015, continue to influence women around the world to this date.

Ms. Jolie announced to the world that she had elective surgery to remove both breasts as a preventive measure. Though she had no cancer, nor signs of disease, she decided to undergo a voluntary double mastectomy as a prophylactic action.[2] She has the gene mutation associated with breast cancer known as the BRCA1 gene, which is a risk factor. In 2015, she followed up her 2013 aggressive decision with another invasive surgery to remove her ovaries. She published her reasoning in the New York Times.[3] Some experts supported Ms. Jolie's choice and hoped it would encourage other women to do the same.[4] She pointed out that women who have a mutated BRCA1 gene have an increased risk for breast and ovarian cancers. Part of her motivation was that her mother died at age fifty-six after a ten-year battle with ovarian cancer. She justified her decision based on statistics on increased risks.

According to the National Cancer Institute (NCI), women with the BRCA1 mutation have a seventy-two percent probability of developing breast cancer and a forty-four percent probability of developing ovarian cancer by age eighty.[5] The overall risk for breast cancer is twelve percent. For ovarian cancer, it is a little under one and a half percent.

HOW MANY BREAST CANCER PATIENTS HAVE BRCA1 MUTATION?

Considering the statistics of how BRCA1 mutation increases cancer risk, one can understand Ms. Jolie's thinking. There is no judgment or criticism here. But let's slow down a minute and think about the consequences of such an action, versus the potential benefits. Are there other statistics that

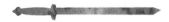

should be considered when contemplating the radical decision to remove both breasts and ovaries? The answer is YES. First, very few women have BRCA1 mutations. Here are the percentages of women with the gene grouped by ethnicity:[6]

Hispanic	3.5%
African American	1.3%
Asian American	0.5%
Ashkenazi Jews	8.3%
Non-Hispanic White	2.2%

Up to ten percent of breast cancers can be attributed to oncogenes.[7] Only five percent of women who have breast cancer have BRCA1 or BRCA2. When considering BRCA1, the mutation Ms. Jolie has, less than five percent of women with breast cancer have that mutated gene. What does this mean?

Ninety-five percent of all breast cancer cases are not caused by the inherited BRCA1 breast cancer gene mutation.

If only five percent of all breast cancer can be attributed to BRCA1 mutation, what is causing ninety-five percent of the other cancers? This is a great question because it brings to light that treating cancer strictly as a genetic disease is not addressing the other factors that cause ninety-five percent of all breast cancer cases. This is not only a problem, it is an enormous opportunity. Cancer must be treated as more than a genetic disease. This is the scientific platform underlying the treatment philosophy of the Oasis of Hope's *Core* and *Enhanced* protocols, which employ a metabolic approach to cancer treatment.

To effectively treat cancer, the first step is to understand how it works. After we explain how cancer starts, develops and spreads, we will begin part two of the book, where we will outline the strategies Oasis of Hope has designed to slow, control, and in many cases, reverse cancer.

Cancer is an opportunistic disease that forms when the immune system underperforms.

HOW CANCER STARTS

It's important to state that every single once of us has mutated cells circulating throughout our bodies. Cancer gets its start with mutations in the DNA. Some of these mutations are inherited from parents, and others are due to environmental factors. Fortunately, God gave humans genes that can repair DNA mutations, and an immune system proficient at targeting abnormal cells, attaching to them, killing them and eliminating them. Having mutated cells does not constitute having cancer. But, abnormal cells can become cancer through hyperplasia—

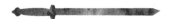

the accelerated cell division of cells that appear normal caused by chronic irritation and other factors; and dysplasia—a rapid build-up of cells that look abnormal, such as moles;[8] and neoplasia—the abnormal and uncontrolled growth of cells that form tumors.[9]

It's essential to understand what factors, in addition to genetic disposition, lead from hyperplasia to dysplasia to neoplasia and then cancer. Cancer is an opportunistic disease. It starts to form when the immune system underperforms for reasons such as illness, chronic, infection and chronic emotional stress.

Cancer stem cells, also known as cancer-initiating cells, have the power to form and sustain tumors.[10] Cancer stem cells have both genetic and metabolic traits that, in large part, have been investigated and identified. The knowledge of cancer genetics and cancer metabolism are the most critical factors for developing anticancer treatments.

Typically, oncogenesis initiates within cells that mutate and reproduce in a chaotic and unorganized fashion. Abnormal cells then begin to form tumors in vital organs or other parts of the anatomy. Cancerous cells are commonly referred to as malignant cells. They thrive even in the absence of oxygen because of their affinity for glucose. When the glucose supply is limited, cancer cells can convert fatty acids into the energy required to multiply.[11] Malignant cells can adapt their metabolism according to the micro-environmental changes around them. Adaptability helps them survive and proliferate, even when cut off from their primary energy source. Because cancer cells reproduce with less metabolic requirements than healthy cells, they can gain strength in numbers and form tumors. Most cancers are diagnosed once a tumor has been formed.

Another way to understand how cancer starts and progresses is to compare and contrast malignant cells with healthy cells. Let's take a closer look.

MALIGNANT CELLS VS. HEALTHY CELLS

There are significant differences between the life of malignant cells and healthy cells:

Reproduction and Development

Normal cells reproduce and develop until the body's need for the specific cells is met. For instance, when skin sustains a scrape or cut, new cells are produced to repair and replace the tissue that sustained the injury. Once the restoration is complete, no more cells are produced. Healthy cells stop reproducing and developing when the body's needs are met.

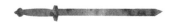

They reproduce only when needed. Malignant cells never put on the brakes. They continuously reproduce abnormally until a tumor is formed, and then they grow the tumor indefinitely. If not dealt with effectively, they will send out cells to develop tumors in other vital organs. Cancer spreading to distant organs is the process called metastasizing. Each type of cancer usually has a specific set of proteins that continue to stimulate the unhealthy reproduction of the abnormal cells through cell division, cell invasion and cell reproduction.

Cell Communication is Different

Healthy cells communicate and interact with each other through cell signaling transduction. They are highly responsive to signals sent from other cells. Through intercellular communication, they know when it is time to reproduce and when it is time to stop growing or reproducing. Malignant cells do not communicate or pass on a signal to stop reproducing.

Cancerous cells are immortal.

Cell Death (Apoptosis)

Normal cells have an expiration date. Programmed cell death, a normal and controlled part of an organism's growth, is called *apoptosis*. As a cell ages, it will eventually die and give way to new replacement cells. Malignant cells never get repaired, nor do they expire when they get old. They are missing the cell death program, which is called "apoptosis." Another way to state it is that cancer cells are immortal. In a healthy cell, there is a protein known as p53, which checks up on the cells. Its primary function is to determine whether a cell is damaged or near its death. If so, it orders the damaged or aged cell to expire. One reason why malignant cells never die is that the p53 protein acts abnormally or does not function.

Cell Cohesion

Healthy cells stick together. Proteins such as laminin make normal cells cohesive. Malignant cells vary in cohesiveness. Many cancerous cells do not cohere well to each other. The improper function of proteins, such as laminin, is one of the factors that can induce cancer cells' spread.[12] Low cell cohesion allows malignant cells to break away from the tissue group and circulate to other parts of the body through the bloodstream and the lymphatic system.[13]

Difference in Appearance

Healthy cells are uniform in size, shape and overall appearance. Malignant cells are present in different shapes

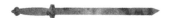

and sizes. They can be larger or smaller than normal cells. The form of malignant cells and their nuclei is abnormal and not well defined.

Extra DNA

The nucleus of a normal cell is smaller and lighter than that of a malignant cell because mutated cells are often polyploid, which means that they carry an excessive amount of DNA.[14] Cancerous polyploidy cells have an additional set of chromosomes, which can be seen by an electron microscope. Some researchers are considering how to use this difference from healthy cells to target cancer cells. Because malignant cells have excess DNA, their nuclei appear larger and darker. The extra number of chromosomes causes abnormal chromosomal arrangement within the cancerous cells.

Cell Maturity Level

When healthy cells mature, they die. In comparison to normal cells, malignant cells grow rapidly and continue reproducing. Because of this rapid reproduction rate, cancerous cells do mature fully. For that reason, they never die. Different maturity levels are referred to as the "grade" of the malignant cells. Level three is the highest grade, and it signifies the most aggressive cancer.

Malignant cells can trick the immune system and stay inside the body forever, unlike normal cells that get eliminated by the immune system once they get damaged. There can be numerous other differences between healthy cells and malignant cells in addition to the primary ones listed above. So here is the million-dollar question:

Is cancer genetic or metabolic?

The answer is...(drum roll)....................... **both**. Cancer is one of the most complex and complicated diseases. It has been affecting humanity since the early civilizations. It is mentioned in the Bible in passages, including Proverbs 12:4 and 2 Timothy 2:17. Over time it has been evolving, mutating and becoming more challenging to treat. Cancer was much easier to treat forty years ago than it is now. Gene mutation may be one reason. Exhaustive research has been conducted to find the origin and cause of cancer and how to treat it. Billions of dollars have been on the genetic analysis of cancer, and annual spending on this research is increasing significantly. Studies on genes have identified many genetic factors that play major roles in cancer's metabolism.

Cancer is both a genetic and a metabolic disease.

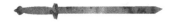

Cancer gene mutations have a significant effect on three major metabolic pathways of the body:

1. Aerobic glycolysis.
2. Glutaminolysis.
3. One-carbon metabolism.

Energy is produced in cells through these metabolic pathways. When affected by cancer gene mutations, the production of massive quantities of amino acids, fatty acids, nucleotides, and other substances occurs instead. The production of these elements instead of energy leads to the rapid growth and division of malignant cells. In other words, genetic factors leverage metabolic factors to either induce or inhibit cancer's proliferation. If genetic factors affect the metabolic traits of normal and abnormal cells, isn't it logical that treatments should be developed to leverage these metabolic traits against cancer?

Well, treating cancer based on metabolic characteristics is not the focus of most pharmaceutical companies. Today, the vast majority of cancer research dollars are spent on treating cancer as a genetic disease. But treating cancer as a genetic disease should not be the only focus. In the past, there was substantial scientific data that cancer is a metabolic disease.

The various aspects of a malignant cell's metabolism can be leveraged to undermine cancer. Imagine how large buildings are imploded. Dynamite is placed in strategic points to weaken the structure inside so that the building falls in on itself when detonated. The metabolic traits could be considered the weak points that we can apply metabolic therapies to so that cancer could fall in on itself.

Treating cancer solely as a genetic disease has several significant disadvantages. Oasis of Hope focuses on the metabolic traits of malignant cells to leverage the weaknesses of cancer overlooked by genetic therapies.

DOWNSIDES TO GENETIC CANCER TREATMENT

Identifying oncogenes and developing drugs that target cancer-causing genes is fascinating. Genetic therapies tempt one to believe that such an approach is the ultimate way to cure cancer. Genetic medicine is so complex and hard to understand that can fall to fantasy thinking an assume it is an advanced medical panacea. The scientific explanation is so mesmerizing and incomprehensible that it cloaks gene therapy in a shroud of seductive mystery. But there are downsides to concluding that cancer is only a genetic disease and should be treated as such.

The main challenges facing gene therapy for cancer are:

1. There is an overwhelming number of cancer-associated genes.
2. The cost of drug development is hyper-inflated.

3. Prices of gene therapies are exorbitant.
4. Cancer gene therapies are not widely approved and available.

Let's take a closer look at these problems. There are one thousand cancer-associated genes that have been identified.[15] There are fewer than fifty cancer targeted therapies approved by the FDA.[16] According to the National Institute of Cancer, new cancer drugs are launching with an annual cost of more than $400,000.00 per patient.[17] Yes, you read that right—Four hundred thousand dollars per patient per year.

Gene therapy will not cure cancer anytime soon.

To date, there are no gene therapies specifically for cancer that are approved and available in the United States; for now. Gene therapies will come soon but would only be accessible to the ultra-rich for many decades to come.[18] Gene therapy is not going to cure cancer anytime soon. Why? Most gene-targeting treatments treat only one cancer-associated gene. But, a person who has cancer may have multiple oncogenes. Imagine if a gene therapy has an annual cost of $400,000.00, the monthly cost would be a little over $33,000.00 per month. If a person had three identified gene mutations, they could have a gene therapy expense of approximately $100,000.00 per month.

UPSIDES OF METABOLIC CANCER TREATMENT

Oasis of Hope's *total care approach* addresses the genetic factors of cancer but focuses on the metabolic impact mutations cause. To better understand the upsides of metabolic cancer treatment, review this table and consider the side-by-side comparison of metabolic therapies with gene therapies.

Metabolic Therapy	Gene Therapy
Available	Not Available
Affordable	Not Affordable
Cancer cell targeted therapy	Cancer cell targeted therapy
Effective	Experimental
In use at Oasis of Hope for nearly sixty years	Still in clinical trials
Will not harm healthy cells	May harm healthy cells

METABOLIC TRAITS OF MALIGNANT CELLS

Leveraging the metabolic traits of cancer cells is the main treatment strategy at Oasis of Hope Hospital. One of the first, and most important, contributions to the explanation of cancer's metabolism was made by the German physician Dr. Otto Heinrich Warburg.

In 1927, Otto Warburg proposed his theory that highlighted cancer cells' unique set of metabolic phenotypes. At the heart of Warburg's theory is aerobic glycolysis. His work demonstrated the abnormal metabolism of tumor cells. Cancer cells convert glucose to lactate while normal cells convert it to pyruvate.[19] This is known as the *Warburg Effect*. The primary reason why cancer cells convert glucose to lactate is that they are hypoxic—very low in oxygen. Cancer cells can thrive and proliferate in an anaerobic environment. This is an important trait of cancer's metabolic phenotype and part of the reason why tumor cells evade apoptosis. [20]

Another important metabolic trait is that malignant cells require two hundred times more glucose to produce energy than normal cells do. This is why Oasis of Hope stresses that sugar (glucose) feeds tumors and we prescribe a diet of foods that are low on the glycemic index. God only knows why so many oncologists discard the importance of nutrition in cancer care. They seem to deny the obvious fact that there are foods that feed cancer and foods that starve cancer. An oncologist cannot intelligently deny cancer's affinity for glucose considering the fact that one of the most important diagnostic tools used by oncologists works precisely based on this fact. When an oncologist prescribes a Positron Emission Tomography (PET

Scan) to a patient, a radio-tracer is injected into a patient. The radio-tracer has small radioactive particles that are detected by the PET Scan. The most common radio-tracer is F-18 fluorodeoxyglucose.

When this glucose solution is injected into the patient. The glucose becomes highly concentrated in the cancer cells and the scan highlights the radioactive material that accumulates in the sugar concentrations. This is how a PET Scan identifies the location, size and shape of tumors.

ONCOMETABOLITES

The emerging research on oncometabolites is underscoring the importance of Otto Warburg's work, and revealing the opportunity to exploit cancer's metabolic traits. In previous paragraphs, we highlighted that malignant cells are hypoxic (low in oxygen). The mitochondrion is the part of a cell that is responsible for the cell's respiration and energy production. Cancer cells have damaged mitochondria, and this leads to the accumulation of metabolites, known as oncometabolites, that activate and oncogenic cascade. Oncometabolites are partly responsible for tumorigenesis.

One of the first oncometabolites discovered was 2-hydroxglutarate. Now, 2-hydroxglutarate is a relatively rare

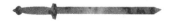

metabolite, which is found in the gliomas. Typically, this substance is known to alter the histone methylation patterns, which then leads to the formation of carcinogenesis in the cancer cells. [21]

After the discovery of 2-hydroxglutarate, many other types of oncometabolites have been identified. Different types of cancers have different oncometabolites. Some cancers have some oncometabolites in common.

Known oncometabolites include fumarate (renal cell carcinoma), succinate (paraganglioma), sarcosine (prostate cancer), glycine (breast cancer), glucose (most cancers), glutamine (myc-dependent cancers), serine (most cancers), asparagine (leukemia), choline (prostate, brain, breast cancer), lactate (most cancers), and polyamines (most cancers). The majority of these oncometabolites originate from aerobic glycolysis, glutaminolysis or one-carbon metabolism.

USING METABOLIC TRAITS FOR DETECTION

Through this discovery of different oncometabolites, it is possible to detect cancer mutations at an early stage just by identifying and looking for the sudden metabolic changes in cell formation. These metabolic changes can be apparent through the changes measured in the levels of acetate, serine, lactate, asparagine, sarcosine, dimethylspermine, betaine or choline in blood, saliva, breath or urine.

In relation to that, it has been identified that almost ninety-five percent of mutated cells originate metabolically and are difficult to discover through genetic screening. Metabolite screening has proved to be faster and more efficient at detecting pre-cancerous cells and malignant cells in early stages.

USING METABOLIC TRAITS FOR TREATMENT

Cancer's metabolic traits offer a vast opportunity to analyze and develop strategies to beat it in a similar way a business develops a plan to beat its competition. A SWOT analysis is a strategic tool used in business to assess the Strengths, Weaknesses, Opportunities and Threats of an organization or business opportunity. This is an efficient, time-saving tool that helps in further processing the organization. In chapter eight, we will show how we use a SWOT analysis to develop a personalized treatment plan.

CONCLUSION

Cancer is both a genetic and metabolic disease. Treating it as a genetic disease could be an effective approach but has some drawbacks including: 1) A tumor may have multiple

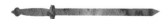

cancer-associated gene mutations, 2) Treatment costs prohibit access to such therapies, and 3) There are no gene therapies for cancer treatment currently available. Cancer's metabolic traits can be leveraged against it. By understanding cancer's metabolic strengths, weakness, opportunities and threats, effective treatment modalities can be developed to undermine cancer and cause it to self-destruct.

In upcoming chapters, we will begin to explain the strategies and treatments we have developed over the past six decades to treat cancer as a metabolic disease. As a teaching tool, each chapter will look through the framework of General Sun Tzu's *The Art of War*.

STORY OF HOPE

Sharon Wiebe • Breast Cancer • 2015

When I was diagnosed with an aggressive stage 2b breast cancer in May of 2015, I was determined to learn all I could about possible treatments before deciding what to do. I attended the "chemo class" at the cancer clinic and spent countless hours researching possibilities. My investigation helped me understand the importance of not harming my body or destroying my immune system when I needed it most. It was during this time that I found the Oasis of Hope website. After learning about their higher than average success rates and their willingness to embrace all healing modalities, I felt hope for the first time.

Dr. Contreras sent me back a treatment plan within two days that included a wide variety of therapies. He explained that they attacked cancer from many different directions and with a wide range of techniques to weaken and eventually overcome its growth, while at the same time, building and strengthening my whole system to help with the fight. This was a very different approach than what was offered in Canada: surgery, chemotherapy and radiation.

From the moment they picked me up at the San Diego airport, I knew I had made the right choice. The kind, supportive care I received, the daily education while sitting in the treatment room, and the bi-weekly meetings with the entire medical team showed me what real medicine should look like. I chose to return for two more immune treatments and after a little over a year, my circulating tumor cell count had gone from off the charts to zero. I have just passed my five-year remission milestone and am happy to say I am feeling great and have no signs of disease.

—Sharon Wiebe
Red Deer, Alberta
Canada

OASIS OF HOPE
HOSPITAL
Stories of Hope

PART TWO

始計

THREE

EVALUATE

Many calculations lead to victory,
and few calculations lead to defeat,
how much more no calculation at all!

—Sun Tzu
The Art of War
Laying Plans

If you fail to prepare, prepare to fail! We can see a great example of this in the famous Bible story of David and Goliath. Goliath failed to prepare for a battle against a skilled shepherd boy. David's preparations were crucial to his victory. This story can truly inspire anyone facing the cancer giant. David killed Goliath with a small pebble. At Oasis of Hope, we like to think of the small stone as an apricot pit—the source of laetrile!

Many lessons can be learned from David and Goliath. Goliath literally lived out the Proverb, "Pride goes before destruction, and a haughty spirit before a fall."[1] He strutted around proudly with great disdain for the Hebrew army. He was taunting and intimidating everyone. Then one, small-for-his-age adolescent, without armor, without a sword, without a spear, took a sling and some smooth stones and caused the prideful, haughty giant to fall! David teaches us several lessons that can be applied to your fight against cancer:

1. Be courageous no matter how large the enemy is.
2. Listen to your positive inner voice and the encouraging words of the Lord.
3. Protect yourself from the negative words and thoughts of others.

Beyond courage, David also teaches a fundamental lesson, which is the focus of this chapter—evaluation. David assessed the situation, sized up the enemy, and evaluated his skills, experiences, weapons and strategies. In a proper assessment, the strengths, weaknesses, opportunities and threats should be identified for both the person and the opponent. David's evaluation could be summed up in a chart like this:

	David	Goliath
Strengths	Experience killing lions and bears. Good with a sling. Faith that God would help him kill Goliath.	Size, strength, highly-trained warrior with countless victories.
Weaknesses	Small in stature. Never gone to war.	Pride. Goliath underestimated David.
Opportunities	Goliath's forehead was not protected.	Goliath could have humbled himself.
Threats	David's brothers didn't believe in him.	Goliath wielded a colossal sword and wore armor.

What was the result of David's evaluation and subsequent execution of his strategy? Read 1 Samuel 17:50 for the answer.

So David triumphed over the Philistine with a sling and a stone; without a sword in his hand he struck down the Philistine and killed him. [2]

In this chapter, we will talk about how to evaluate the enemy —cancer. We won't stop there because a proper evaluation includes looking at oneself closely. In our experience, most patients unknowingly aid and abet the progression and spread of cancer. Sun Tzu's first strategy in *The Art of War* is "Laying Plans." In this strategy, he stresses that the general who makes many calculations in the temple will later have victory out on the battlefield.[4] Evaluation is the beginning of the calculation process.

When evaluating yourself, it's essential to consider multiple factors. For example, is there anything in your home environment that could help the growth and spread of cancerous cells? Does your diet starve or feed cancer? Are there other factors in your lifestyle that promote cancer?

When evaluating cancer, it's important to point out that the same type of cancer will behave differently in each person. It's critical to evaluate each patient individually. There are numerous assessment tools to evaluate cancer. Before we go further, let's share some definitions from the *NCI Dictionary of Cancer Terms.*[4]

TERMINOLOGY

Benign
> Not cancerous. Benign tumors may grow larger but do not spread to other parts of the body. Also called *nonmalignant*.

Malignant
> Cancerous. Malignant cells can invade and destroy nearby tissue and spread to other parts of the body.

Diagnosis
> The process of identifying a disease, condition, or injury from its signs and symptoms. A health history, physical exam, and tests, such as blood tests, imaging tests, and biopsies, may help make a diagnosis.

Prognosis
> The likely outcome or course of a disease, the chance of recovery or recurrence.

As you are making calculated decisions about how to undermine cancer, the terms above should be understood. You may have heard your doctors use them when they talk about your case. If the doctor said that the results of a biopsy were benign, the tissue sample that was removed and analyzed was not cancerous. In general, this would be excellent news, but note that other tests should be done to confirm the results. Though benign cells are not cancerous and won't spread to other organs, in some cases, they can be life-threatening. Some

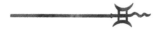

benign tumors grow and exert pressure on surrounding organs. Benign brain tumors can be dangerous and sometimes are inoperable.

If your doctor has used the term "malignant," the mass is cancer. A diagnosis will be given when the evaluation of lab tests, radiological tests, medical history, physical exam and pathology reports provide enough information to make a determination. When an oncologists gives a prognosis, it is a probability of recovery based on statistics gathered from similar cases. It is as estimate and should therefore be looked at as a guideline, not a definitive fact for the individual patient.

CANCER TYPES SIMILARITIES & DIFFERENCES

Some patients ask questions such as, "If I have breast cancer, why am I taking the same hyperthermia treatment a prostate cancer patient is taking?" Because the metabolism of malignant cells is the common denominator for all cancers, Oasis of Hope patients are given the same *Core* therapies regardless of cancer type. Each protocol is personalized, however. We administer cancer-specific targeting therapies unique for each patient. We will share more in chapters later on in the book.

Though all cancer types share common metabolic traits, it is imperative to evaluate each patient individually. Each tumor has different traits and evolutions. Cancer is a "family of diseases." As stated before, though cancers have similarities, they also have differences, just like siblings in a family. For cells to be classified as cancer, they will all share phenotypes. But, each cancer type has different observable characteristics. For example, cancer of the breast itself is divided into various categories depending on different variables each breast cancer may exhibit. There are mutations within the same category and types of tumors, which is another factor when designing the treatment protocol.

INTEGRATIVE CANCER TREATMENT

To determine how to treat a patient effectively, we conduct a thorough evaluation of the data we collect through a physical examination, medical history, laboratory work, radiological studies and biopsies. We identify how aggressive the tumor is and how fast it is growing and if it is spreading. We formulate, customize and dose the therapies individually based on the medical information we obtain during the evaluation of each patient's case.

Though the differences in our treatment protocols may be subtle, we continuously make slight adjustments depending on our patients' individual needs and responses to the regimen.

Lifestyle medicine may be slow-acting, but it can lead to longer-lasting results than drug therapies.

SLOW-GROWING TUMORS

If a patient has a slow-growing tumor, we can be gentle and utilize diet and lifestyle with very few pharmaceuticals. Lifestyle medicine using is slow acting, but it can lead to long-lasting results. Lifestyle medicine using is slow acting, but it can lead to long lasting results.

AGGRESSIVE CANCERS

When cancer is highly aggressive, we integrate conventional therapies with lifestyle and natural therapies. Most patients that come to Oasis of Hope are looking for alternatives to chemotherapy, radiation and surgery. Still, our board-certified licensed clinical and surgical oncologists evaluate each case to determine if there could be any benefit to using some conventional therapies. We are not against conventional cancer treatments; we are against the ineffective use of conventional oncology that easily harms the quality of life. Conventional treatment can be highly useful to buy the time a patient needs to reap the benefits of our gentle immune building therapies. In most cases, conventional treatments are only helpful in the short term. For long-lasting results, we utilize natural therapies that, though they require time to take effect, have a profound effect on the tumor's lifecycle and the patient's quality of life.

Conventional therapies may be productive initially, but the benefits obtained fade fast. Natural therapies take effect slower, but their benefits are far-reaching and much more substantial, especially for long term success. Alternative cancer treatment is necessary because of chemotherapies' limitations. To understand how limited chemotherapy, is, an extensive comparative study reviewed survival data from the US and Australia. It concluded, "The overall contribution of curative and adjuvant cytotoxic chemotherapy to 5-year survival in adults was estimated to be 2.3% in Australia and 2.1% in the USA."[5] We don't unilaterally dismiss chemotherapy because it can buy time for slower acting alternative therapies to work. A patient with a prognosis of three months may need some chemotherapy to quickly reduce tumor mass and provide time to respond to our natural therapies. Our integrative use of

conventional and natural therapies is beneficial in some aggressive, fast-growing tumors.

To integrate therapies, we conduct a thorough evaluation that takes multiple factors into consideration. We create a tumor profile based on its growth rate, aggressiveness and genetic makeup. We evaluate the tumor's cellular characteristics and assess it by its type and stage. The stage is a way to catalog how advanced the tumor is and determine its prognosis. The stage is not an indicator of a tumor's growth rate. For example, a localized tumor that is half a centimeter in size is not an advanced-stage. Even if it is aggressive and fast-growing, and has an unfavorable genetic profile, the probability of cure is high. Its size and the fact that it has not spread make it early-stage cancer. However, the same tumor that spreads to another organ, or grows to be more than three centimeters in size, is an advanced stage and is more difficult to treat.[6]

Chapter thirteen will look at how to treat cancer effectively by making adjustments for the stage. Now, let's see how a cancer type and stage are determined during evaluation. If a patient has breast cancer, and a mass is also detected in the lung, the patient has stage IV breast cancer. The size of the tumor is not the factor determining the stage. It is stage IV because the primary tumor has spread to a distant organ. Another way to state it is that the patient has breast cancer with lung metastases. Cancer that has metastasized is also referred to as "Advanced-stage metastatic cancer." One more thing to note about stage IV cancer is that there is no further staging or sub-staging after stage IV.

Let's use the same example of breast cancer with lung metastases. It's not lung cancer because the primary tumor of the breast has spread to the lung. If a biopsy of the mass in the lung were taken, breast cancer cells would be found. A metastasis is when cells break off from the primary tumor and spread to form tumors in a different organ or tissue. Evaluation is critical because there are cases in which cancer is found in more than one organ, but there are two different primary cancers. Though rare, a patient may have two types of cancer at the same time. However, it is more common that a patient has one primary cancer that spreads to other organs. As oncologists, it is imperative to get the diagnosis right during evaluation to craft the best treatment for each patient.

MISDIAGNOSIS

We always verify a diagnosis and never take the word of a doctor from another treatment center. Our team reviews and repeats whatever tests deemed necessary to confirm, or update,

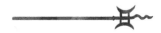

the diagnosis. Over the years, we have found that between five percent and ten percent of our patients have been misdiagnosed. In some cases, the patient didn't even have cancer. In other cases, the diagnosis was an incorrect type or stage of cancer.

We are alarmed when we find a misdiagnosis, and the patient has taken treatment based on the error. Can you imagine being given the wrong chemotherapy? This further underscores why a proper evaluation is essential in developing strategies to best combat cancer.

The consequences of a misdiagnosis can be deadly. For example, we have seen a case where the oncologists had done a mastectomy, but a follow-up PET scan revealed that the breast cancer had already metastasized to the liver. One objective of a mastectomy is to prevent the spread of cancer, but if it has already metastasized, a mastectomy may not be the best option.

Below is the case study of one of our more recent patients, who came to us with a misdiagnosis. His misdiagnosis could have very well proved to be fatal. Fortunately, our evaluation corrected the diagnosis and put him on the correct treatment regimen. The patient's name is not included to protect privacy.

CASE STUDY

Male patient, age forty-five, presenting with a diagnosis of prostate cancer, of which treatment is being provided. His complaint is a continual progression of cancer. He comes to us in a very poor general condition. He cannot eat, and movement is restricted, due tremendous abdominal pain. His diagnosis of prostate cancer, which is currently being treated, is showing minimal response to therapies.

As soon as he arrives at our hospital, we see that he has had a comprehensive medical exploration. We also notice that many of his symptoms are not typical of prostate cancer. We decide to do a PET scan. The results that we get are astounding. According to the PET scan results, there is no tumor activity in the prostate. However, he has an enormous tumor in the upper abdomen. Our radiologist reports that the primary tumor is in the pancreas. The patient had been wrongly treated for prostate cancer before coming to Oasis of Hope. How was that mistake made when the PET scan showed cancer in the abdomen, not the prostate or pelvic area?

After determining that he was misdiagnosed, we do several tumor markers. We do not opt for a biopsy because his general health is too poor to withstand invasive procedures. The prostate-specific antigen (PSA) tumor marker confirms that there is no sign of prostate cancer. The CA-19 cancer marker returns positive, which further supports a diagnosis of pancreatic cancer.

Here we have a young man whose life is in jeopardy because he has been treated for six months for the wrong disease. Shockingly, he was misdiagnosed and treated for the wrong type of cancer by an oncologist at a major treatment center in Los Angeles, California. It's incomprehensible

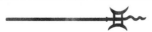

how such a big blunder could have happened. Our best guess is that it was a typing error from a transcriptionist. More than likely, the oncologist said, "pancreas," but the transcription came back saying, "prostate." We came up with this explanation because we can't accept that a doctor would make such a big mistake. The error had been perpetuated for months, and the patient had been sent home to die. Ordering a PET scan upon his arrival to Oasis of Hope saved his life.

The error in the above case could have been corrected by conducting another evaluation when the patient's condition worsened, and cancer did not respond to treatment. Because of cases like this, we double-check all diagnoses and conduct further detailed evaluations of our own.

However, it does not mean that we blindly have patients repeat batteries of tests. In our evaluation, we validate results from other centers. For example, if a patient has a recent PET scan, we won't send them to do another one. Quality of life is paramount for our patients. We don't want to exhaust our patients' energy and finances on unnecessary tests.

ARE BENIGN TUMORS DANGEROUS?

Some people think that benign tumors do not warrant concern. But the word "benign" does not equate to non-harmful in every case. There is still a tumor that could be dangerous.

Though the risk can be less because it is not malignant, a benign tumor may present problems, even life-threatening problems. The prime example of a benign tumor being dangerous is when the tumor is in the brain.

Most benign tumors are not life-threatening, but may still need to be removed. For example, a benign tumor in the kidney may affect renal function. Surgical removal of the tumor could restore normal kidney function. Though the tumor is not cancerous and will not spread, it has to be removed. If left untreated, it will impede the kidney's function. In the worst-case scenario, the benign tumor could continue to grow, cause kidney failure and possibly lead to death.

As mentioned previously in the chapter, a benign tumor in the brain can be extremely dangerous. It can grow and affect brain function or induce a coma. Because benign tumors don't respond to chemotherapy, the only treatment option is surgery. Removing a brain tumor is a delicate process, and not all brain tumors are operable. A patient with a benign brain tumor doesn't have cancer, yet the prognosis may still be poor.

BENIGN CANCER?

The term "cancer" is only used for malignant tumors. However, a doctor may refer to cancer as *benign* or *indolent,*

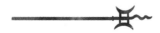

meaning that it is growing very slowly and is not life-threatening. For these types of tumors, doctors make use of the process of watchful waiting. Though it is cancer, it behaves as if it were benign and does not need intervention. The doctor will not say that you have a benign tumor; he may refer to it as benign if it is very slow-growing and not likely to need treatment.

Healthy lifestyle behaviors undermine cancer.

EVALUATING LIFESTYLE

Lifestyle behaviors can promote cancer. They can also undermine cancer. We emphasize lifestyle because it is the most potent agent that slows or reverses cancer growth in the long run. It may be the number one factor in sustaining a long-term victory over cancer. It is paramount that we teach patients what lifestyle changes to make and encourage them to adopt the healthy habits essential to prolonging their lives. Changes in lifestyle may be the hardest ask we make to our patients. Nobody likes to change. We avoid pressuring people, and opt for continuous education, motivation and coaching. We aren't bullies, we are cheerleaders. We work hard to cheer our patients and their families on to success. We also try to focus on the most important lifestyle factors and disregard the lessor factors to avoid overwhelming our patients.

Oasis of Hope promotes healthy lifestyle changes in nutrition, exercise, stress management, home environment, and smoking and drinking cessation.

OASIS OF HOPE LIFESTYLE FOCUS AREAS

Food

We teach what foods heal and what foods harm. We will go in depth about food and our nutrition program later as nutrition is one of the most significant lifestyle factors. We will share about the importance of the glycemic index when eating to fight cancer.

Movement

The body was designed to move. Movement is the only way the lymph system will work. Movement increases circulation, detoxification and oxygenation. We are use the word "movement" because "exercise" is a swear word to some people.

Stress Management

Stress could likely be equal to nutrition as the number one lifestyle factor leading to cancer and heart disease. We help our patients evaluate their stress levels and teach them how to manage stress through relaxation techniques and spirituality. Laughter therapy is an effective stress management and immune-stimulating interventions we

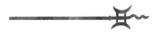

promote.[7] We occasionally provide laughter therapy sessions at Oasis of Hope. Our founder was the first to do this therapy at our hospital, and laughter is the most potent anti-stress agent we have identified to date.

Home Environment

We teach our patients about creating a home environment that diminishes the use of carcinogenic products such as chemical cleaning agents. It is vital to have a smoke-free environment as second-hand smoke is deadly.

Tobacco-Free

All types of tobacco use must become a part of your past. Quitting smoking is the number one lifestyle change a person can do to prevent cancer.

It also is critical not to vape if you are fighting cancer. Chewing tobacco is also dangerous as it is linked to cancers in the mouth.

Alcohol

Drinking any type of alcohol is a documented cancer risk. The risk outweighs the heart-protective benefits of red wine's resveratrol. Abstaining from alcohol—wine, beer and spirits—is best.

Evaluating a patient's eating habits, physical movement, health-harming habits and home environment is an integral part of our treatment program. A thorough assessment can bring to light issues that need attention. We recently had a patient with lung cancer who had never smoked a cigarette in his life. When we asked about his work, he shared that he had been working as a bartender for the previous fifteen years. Exposure to second-hand smoke for eight hours a day over fifteen years resulted in cancer.

There are many lifestyle factors that we need to evaluate and recommend positive changes. If a patient likes to garden, we recommend not using cancer-causing chemicals, such as *Roundup*,[8] and using organic pesticide-free gardening techniques instead. In some cases, like the bartender, a change of occupation may be in order.   In some cases, like the bartender, a change of occupation may be in order.

We had another patient who was shocked by his cancer diagnosis because he had never had any health problems before. A few years before his diagnosis, his mother had developed cancer. He moved in with her as her caregiver. That's when he developed lung cancer. His sister went to live there and take care of both of them. Would you believe that she also developed cancer? We advised them to have the house tested by electricians. It turned out that the house was located beneath high voltage power lines. It also tested positive for high levels of radon, a radioactive gas emitted from the soil. They immediately moved to our patient's home. According to the National Cancer Institute, two percent to four percent of all lung cancer deaths could be prevented by lowering radon

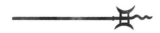

exposure.[9] According to the Environmental Protection Agency (EPA), one in fifteen homes have radon levels higher than the EPA action level. This is another powerful example of why evaluating a patient's lifestyle is critical to providing cancer treatment.

Wellness in the soul and spirit is an integral part of cancer recovery.

HOLISTIC EVALUATION

Whereas conventional oncologists tend to make the destruction of a tumor their singular focus, we know that lifestyle, including a patient's environment, is critical to generate long-lasting results. We include evaluation of the patient's emotional and spiritual health too. Oncologists may consider emotional and spiritual wellbeing to be subjective. But we subscribe to the evidence in studies that point to an emotional component to cancer.[10] Wellness in the soul and spirit is an integral part of the full recovery of our patients.

Our doctor, specialized in palliative care, leads our counseling team that provides group and individual sessions designed to manage stress and work through unresolved emotional issues. We provide a safe place and a path to resolve emotional wounds from the past. Our therapies for the body may work without doing the emotional and spiritual part of our treatment. Still, patients that participate in our education and ministry activities will undoubtedly gain an advantage.

People find profound peace when they resolve to look for wins beyond life extension.

Most assuredly, cancer is a serious issue and no laughing matter. But we need to combat distress because cancer feeds on fear and anxiety. We will expand on the physiological processes triggered by fear later in the book. Now, let us underline the importance of managing the anxiety associated with cancer. Laughter therapy is one way we invite our patients to take a vacation away from distressing thoughts of cancer. We also coach them through the grieving steps of denial, anger, sadness, acceptance and resolve. Resolve does not mean that the patient has decided to fight cancer no matter what. Resolve is closely tied to surrender. People in the "resolve" phase in the fight against cancer find profound peace because they look for wins beyond life extension. They resolve to fill days with meaningful exchanges with God and others. They resolve to forgive others and themselves. They decide to fill their lives with love, joy,

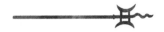

peace, patience, kindness, goodness, faithfulness, gentleness and self-control. They let those fruits spill over into the lives of people around them.

It is common for patients to be in the grief stages of denial or anger when they first arrive at Oasis of Hope. When we see patients progress to the point that they can say, "Yes, I have cancer. It is happening to me. I am going to enjoy my life to the fullest regardless," then we know that the patient is positioned to have the best chance of recovery.

Spirituality helps a person through the phases of acceptance and resolve. Knowing where eternity will be spent helps a person accept each day on earth as a gift from God to be enjoyed and cherished without losing the day to fear about the future. Being free from the fear of death brings joy to the life you have, no matter how long it lasts. Spiritual fortitude bolsters emotional health. Good emotional health enhances healing in the body.

Evaluation is vital for every aspect of our treatment design to support total health–body mind and spirit.
—Dr. Ernesto Contreras, Sr.

MULTIDISCIPLINARY TEAM

We believe that natural health practitioners should be a part of everyone's medical team. But, we also know the importance of having an oncologist on the team as well. At Oasis of Hope, each patient benefits from the care of a multidisciplinary team comprised of a clinical oncologist, surgical oncologist, pathologist, hematologist-oncologist, internist, family medicine practitioner, a medical doctor specialized in oncology counseling, nutritionist and psychologist. Our pastor provides spiritual support. Our team looks at each patient's case from different perspectives, making the evaluation comprehensive and multi-dimensional. Every week, the team meets and goes through every case. Team members weigh in, so the patient benefits from the experience and knowledge of various specialists. The team input facilitates undermining cancer with synergistic strategies. Each patient is assigned an attending physician responsible for daily managing and monitoring of treatment. Patient education is another responsibility of the attending physician.

CONCLUSION

Dr. Ernesto Contreras, Sr. established the importance of a thorough evaluation of a patient's physical, spiritual, emotional

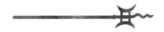

and environmental health. He understood that a good evaluation, or the lack of one, could make the difference between an effective treatment and a poor outcome. His military training taught him to never go into battle without a comprehensive assessment of the enemy and a detailed analysis of the battleground. His medical training affirmed that conviction.

Before Dr. Contreras, Sr. became an oncologist, he specialized in pathology and spent many years evaluating tissue samples. He mastered the skill of evaluation. As he moved into oncology, he never disregarded the necessity and power of evaluation. A thorough assessment identifies the variables, essential data and information needed to develop an effective plan of attack. A multidisciplinary team is key to achieving a comprehensive evaluation.

Story of Hope
Susan Vernon • Stage III Breast Cancer • 2016

What I thought was going to be my usual yearly mammogram, turned into a diagnosis of stage three breast cancer. I found myself in a place of confusion and despair. After a second opinion, I was overwhelmed. The thought of conventional chemo and radiation was terrifying. It made no sense to me to destroy everything good in my body in order to kill the bad. I prayed for another way. I was given the name of Dr. Contreras. After reading about the hospital, I felt it was the place for me to receive treatment. I went for my first visit to Oasis of Hope Hospital in January of 2016. It changed my life! They treat cancer from every angle: Medically, physically, mentally, and spiritually. They have years of experience and success in treating cancer in a way that is kind and gentle to the patient. You learn so much about all the latest research and treatments designed not only to kill cancer, but also to restore health. Nutrition is a big focus and they teach you how to eat to maintain a strong immune system. During meal times, you get amazing food and are able to connect with the other patients. This is a healing process and many friendships are formed out of these encounters. My spiritual needs were also met with as much diligence as my physical and medical needs. This was very important to me.

On April 27th, 2016 I went for my third visit for treatment. During my consultation with Dr. Contreras, he told me I was in total remission! Today, I am well, remain cancer free, and live a normal life. I continue with a healthy lifestyle and continue on my daily protocol. I'm so glad I chose Oasis of Hope as my place for treatment."

—Susan Vernon
Cleveland, TN
United States

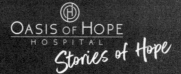

作戰

FOUR

PLAN THE ATTACK

In war, let your great objective be victory.

—Sun Tzu
The Art of War
Waging War

I had the opportunity to present our treatment methodology and results at a cancer conference in Canada some years ago. I confidently explained how we effectively combine alternative therapies, such as high dose Vitamin C infusions and Ozone, with low dose metronomic chemotherapy. During the question and answer period, an indignant oncologist grilled me. He raised his voice on the microphone, asking, "So what kind of medicine do you practice if you are using both alternative and conventional cancer treatments?" My answer was simple and to the point. "I practice good medicine."

The oncologist was not impressed with the short answer, so I explained further. I told him, and the audience of physicians, that many practitioners are passionate about their treatments. In contrast, we are passionate about our patients' quality of life. Both alternative and conventional doctors can be dogmatic about a specific approach to cancer treatment. Alternative doctors want to juice away disease and are at a loss when the green stuff isn't enough. Conventional doctors want to chemo or radiate cancer and throw in the towel cancer comes back.

Oasis of Hope doesn't promote one type of treatment, we promote our patients' wellness.

At Oasis of Hope, we don't practice alternative or conventional medicine, we practice good medicine. We define good medicine as the most effective least aggressive treatment. It is evidence-based and provides maximum therapeutic benefits with minimal side effects. We don't promote specific types of therapies; we promote our patients' wellness.

To us, **it's not what** treatment we offer that is the most critical variable. **It is why** we offer a specific treatment **and how** we plan to use the treatment. In general, maximum-dose chemotherapy offers minimal benefit. But minimal-dose

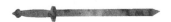

chemotherapy offers maximum benefits. Low-dose chemo doesn't provoke heavy side effects, and it can work really well in combination with natural therapies. Green juice won't cure cancer, but it will boost the immune system. An optimally functioning immune system will repel and eradicate pathogens and foreign molecules.[1] It will also fight cancer better than one that has been demolished by aggressive chemotherapy.

GOOD MEDICINE MUST BE PLANNED

To provide good medicine to our patients, we develop individual treatment plans designed to undermine cancer and promote physical, emotional and spiritual health. Our plan of attack is comprehensive. We don't merely read medical textbooks and prescribe whatever the pharmaceutical companies tell us to. We don't let insurance companies make treatment decisions based on what they approve for reimbursement or deny. No. We evaluate our patients. We analyze the latest published clinical studies. We tap into the wisdom our medical team has garnered over the last fifty-seven years treating tens of thousands of patients. Then we generate a plan of attack to use as a crucial weapon in a patient's fight against cancer. Developing a treatment plan is the next step after a complete evaluation of a patient's lifestyle factors, emotional well-being and disease progression. Our plan of attack incorporates care for a patient's body, mind and spirit.

The treatment plan also considers how aggressive the cancer is and its genetic profile. We take all of the variables mentioned above into account. They are contemplated and addressed to best position our patients for success in the battle against cancer. As can be learned in Sun Tzu's *The Art of War*, everyone has strengths and limitations. The key is to develop a plan of attack that maximizes strengths and compensates for limitations. It is also advantageous for us to design a plan that our patients will comply with happily.

Oasis of Hope plans of attack incorporate care for patients' bodies, minds and spirits.

RESPECTING A PATIENT'S WISHES

When planning treatment, we honor the wishes of our patients. If a patient is open to alternative therapies, we incorporate them into the treatment plan. If a patient is open to conventional therapies, we may recommend low-dose chemotherapy. When a patient is adamantly against using conventional therapies, we recommend alternatives. We

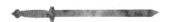

educate our patients on treatment options because there are pros and cons of opting out of all conventional therapy in favor of alternatives only. Take the case or our patient Burga Ratti, from Germany. She came to Oasis of Hope thirty-three years ago. She had deep convictions about what treatments to take and what therapy options were utterly unacceptable. Burga's testimony is amazing, inspiring and compelling. Burga was diagnosed with breast cancer, and simultaneously found out she was pregnant with her second child. Though she was from Germany, she and her family were living in Colorado at the time.

Her oncologist strongly recommended that she have a therapeutic abortion since the hormonal and immune environments of pregnancy favor cell growth, helping cancer proliferate. Burga prayed to the Holy Spirit and decided one hundred percent against the abortion. She sought an alternative doctor, which brought her to Dr. Ernesto Contreras, Sr. He agreed to treat her after her baby was born. Nine months later, she gave birth to a healthy boy who is now in his thirties. Then she started treatment at Oasis of Hope.

Alternative medicine, and the lifestyle changes she made, kept cancer in check for over three decades. Burga's experience helps explain how we design a plan of attack that respects a patient's desires, needs and beliefs. Because of the plan, her baby was born, and Burga added thirty-three years to her life before she went to heaven in July of 2020. Her beautiful testimony and smile will forever be etched in our hearts, and our documentary series *Healthy Long Life*. She was a great health advocate. It is fitting that she is in the documentary series with her heroes like Dr. Caldwell Esselstyn, Jr., T. Colin Campbell, PhD, Dr. Michael Greger and Dr. Dean Ornish.

For Burga, it was essential to have her child be born healthy first, and then add as many years to her life as possible. Over her life extension of three decades, she became a health coach and helped many people live in health. It was partly because Dr. Ernesto Contreras, Sr. was willing to work with Burga's wishes. Her success was mostly due to her determination and discipline.

Most oncology specialists have an ***it's my way or the highway*** attitude. Hospital policies and medical protocols are neither flexible nor negotiable. Many patients have told us how their oncologists have nearly bullied them into treatments. Some patients have been discharged from care because they don't wholly accept a doctor's recommendations. Doctors' all or nothing attitude is most likely based on the fear of being sued for negligence. We don't force treatments on patients because they will not be effective if the patient doesn't want them.

It is vital to win the war on cancer in the patient's mind and heart, not just the body.

PRINCIPLES & DESIRED OUTCOMES

There are many effective cancer killers available for use, but we are selective based on our treatment principles and the patient's desired outcome. Again, considering Burga's case, her priority was not to harm the unborn baby. Chemotherapy was ruled out during her pregnancy. Her desired outcome was to have a healthy baby, and then do her best to survive cancer. She opted for alternative cancer treatment once the baby was born. Her choices, with the support of Oasis of Hope, helped her manage cancer and enjoy a productive life.

We follow our guiding principles and do not offer therapies that would harm our patients, or that we wouldn't take ourselves if we had the same illness. We design therapy protocols to help patients survive and thrive. Our approach is very different than standard oncology, where many chemotherapy protocols take a patient to the brink of death. Chemotherapy is given in cycles to give a patient time to recover from the toxicity. Some protocols require a quarantine following treatment because the patient's immune system is destroyed, and the patient could not survive even the common cold after cancer treatment. It's no wonder that people seek alternatives at Oasis of Hope.

Success is when a patient lives longer than expected and enjoys a high quality of life.

Before starting any treatment, or making any modifications, we always weigh the potential benefits of a treatment option against the cost to the patient's quality of life. Our definition of success is not when a tumor is destroyed, and a patient survives. Success is when a patient lives longer with a high quality of life. We had a family member who was being treated by an oncologist in Southern California. He had her on a chemo protocol that was so brutal, that she told him she would rather die than continue the regimen. That is an example of a treatment that we would never recommend. Aggressive treatments that have no regard for the patient's quality of life have one desired outcome: eradicating cancer.

Oasis of Hope treatment outcome goals include:
- Adding as many months and years to a patient's life as possible.
- Improving a patient's quality of life.
- Boosting a patient's immune system.
- Slowing, controlling cancer and reversing cancer when possible.
- Shielding against a recurrence.
- Helping a patient find peace and emotional healing.
- Helping a patient increase spiritual wellness.
- Educating a patient on an optimal lifestyle so they can share it with their family members and improve their lives.

Considering our principles and desired outcomes, we design a specific plan of attack based on cancer's behavior. When the cancer is not aggressive, the treatment plan can utilize natural therapies, that are simple and elegant. In complicated cases, our treatment plan is going to be more complex and comprehensive. In every case, instead of working against cancer and cornering it, we work for the patient to help them undermine cancer. Our treatment approach is like jujitsu and aikido. In those styles of martial arts, the fighter uses his opponent's force, momentum and bodyweight against them. When the opponent throws a punch, the defender uses the aggressor's momentum and the bodyweight behind it to cause the opponent to fall. In aikido, a fighter doesn't strike the opponent to knock them over. The fighter evades an incoming punch, grabs the opponent's hand and pulls them to the ground in the direction they were already going. The defender steps out of the way and lets the power of the strike pass by. Force is added in the same direction the punch is going. With the momentum of the punch meeting no resistance, the opponent is easily dragged to the ground. The Oasis of Hope's plan of attack is like aikido. We invite cancerous cells to harm themselves with their own force.

There are many things we need to consider in the plan of attack to be successful. Some treatments do not attack cancer directly. Instead, we undermine and weaken cancer's strongholds. We take away the foundations of cancer to help it fall. Our treatment goal is to topple cancer without the patient toppling over with it. Our approach to fighting cancer includes strategies that have resulted in survival rates second to none. In some cases, we go full-blown against the tumor, or surgically remove it. In cases where a direct attack is used, an effective plan must include therapies that hit from other angles.

When fighting cancer, it takes numerous battles to win the war.

An excellent military plan of attack doesn't only focus on the battle. It also makes preparations for winning the war. When fighting cancer, it takes numerous battles to win the war. A thorough evaluation and a plan of attack are necessary. In our plan of attack, we have short-term strategies addressing the current battle against the disease. We implement medium-term

and long-term game plans to diminish the probability of recurrence. We fight to prevent cancer from coming back more viciously.

Standard chemotherapy focuses on the present and attacks to destroy the tumor. At Oasis of Hope, we focus on the long-term. We follow up with our patients for at least five years after their initial treatments. That is tremendous for a patient to know that we are committed to them for the long run.

A MULTIPRONGED APPROACH

A robust plan of attack evaluates and leverages the strengths, weaknesses, opportunities and threats (SWOT) of a patient's case. After analyzing the SWOT of a patient's case, we create a plan of attack, including therapies that address the different aspects of cancer. Sun Tzu's principle of indirect attacks has shown us that an all-out direct attack on cancer will not improve a patient's prognosis and quality of life. Sun Tzu taught to never corner an enemy because when cornered, the enemy can see no escape. If an enemy feels trapped, it will become extremely dangerous. It will fight whole-heartedly with no concern for self-preservation because it knows it is on a suicide mission. The enemy will start taking as many lives with them as possible. It is similar when the focus of cancer treatment is a shock and awe full-on attack. Cancer may look like it is losing, but it will become chemoresistant and come back stronger and more difficult to beat back. We will expand on tackling resistance in chapter twelve.

We developed our multi-prong approach to attack cancer from many different angles. A direct attack strikes cancer at its strongest point. A multi-prong attack, based on the SWOT evaluation, undermines cancer's weak points to make it collapse in on itself.

HDIVC & Amygdalin
work like natural non-toxic chemotherapies.

Our multi-pronged approach considers many different factors and employs a combination of therapies. In general, our strategy will include a direct attack on cancer at a strategic moment. Unlike conventional treatments, our direct attack uses therapies that do not destroy the patient's immune system. Our treatments restore a patient's immune system. Our direct attack includes high dose IV Vitamin C (HDIVC) and amygdalin (Vitamin B17). They are two of the best natural anti-tumor agents, according to scientific literature. Even the National

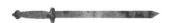

Cancer Institute has published studies that confirm that HDIVC[2] and amygdalin (laetrile)[3] improve patients' quality of life and diminish adverse side effects associated with cancer. They can debilitate cancer in a similar way that chemotherapy does while not provoking unfavorable side effects. We like to think of them as natural non-harmful chemotherapies because of their therapeutic actions.

Depending on the growth and aggressiveness of a tumor, we may rotate in other therapies. We use anti-tumor agents that exploit cancer's metabolic traits. We leverage a tumor's vulnerability to oxidative stress. We have several treatments that increase the stress of oxidation on malignant cells. Once again, high dose intravenous Vitamin C comes into play because it attacks the tumor directly by converting into the oxidative agent peroxide. It also increases a cancer cell's response to other therapies. In other words, it is both a direct and an adjuvant therapy. It brings down the cancer cells' ability to resist other therapies or recur after treatment.

**Oasis of Hope administers natural
immune-boosting agents to fight cancer.**

One of cancer's strengths is its ability to mutate to become chemoresistant. We proactively employ therapies that lower cancer's resistance to future treatment. We pre-condition patients with Ozone to increase the tumors' oxygen levels and facilitate Vitamin C's conversion into peroxide. Ozone potentiates Vitamin C to create an environment that is hostile to the tumor. We also administer natural immune-boosting agents to fight cancer. Immunotherapy is a significant part of our plan of attack. About sixty percent to seventy percent of our therapy is focused on immune system stimulation. In a war analogy, we fortify the local army. We build the army inside—the immune cancer-fighting cells–and get it back in the fight, even when chemotherapy previously demolished it. These strategies are aimed at undermining cancer.

CUTTING OFF SUPPLY LINES

Using another war analogy, we have specific therapies that cut off supply lines to tumors. In World War II, Air Force sorties would fly out to bomb bridges and railways so that the enemy couldn't get the resources needed to survive and advance the war effort. We have several elements that can impede and disrupt the channels that feed the tumor. We utilize both natural therapies and pharmaceuticals that inhibit the

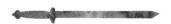

formation of new blood vessels. Tumors must form many new blood vessels to get the supplies they need to multiply, grow and spread. Angiogenesis is the process of new blood vessel formation.[4] Amygdalin and other natural therapies inhibit angiogenesis.

Vascular endothelial growth factor (VEGF) is the main protein required for new blood vessel generation. Using natural VEGF-targeting angiogenesis inhibitors is an essential part of the plan of attack we develop for our patients. We use nutrients to inhibit VEGF. A benefit of fish oil supplementation is the antagonism of VEGF's pro-angiogenic effect. Fish oil can reduce endothelial expression of the Flt-1 receptor for VEGF.[5,6] We also use glycine because its anti-angiogenic action may promote an antioxidant effect that down-regulates VEGF signaling in endothelial cells.[7,8,9]

A real mainstay at Oasis of Hope is EGCG from green tea. EGCG exerts an anti-angiogenic effect. Many studies find that it suppresses VEGF expression and signaling.[10,11,12,13,14,15]

We are currently researching the use of phycocyanobilin to inhibit NADPH oxidase. NADP boosts VEGF activity in endothelial cells. Phycocyanobilin could exert an antioxidant effect.[16,17] Another reason why we use metronomic chemotherapy is that it can also produce anti-angiogenic effects. [18]

FOR THE HEARTS & MINDS OF OUR PATIENTS

As we have mentioned, our treatments go beyond medication administration and natural therapies provided in the form of tablets, food or infusions. Monday through Friday, we provide education about treatments and lifestyle habits that can help beat cancer and protect against recurrence. We teach what boosts the immune system and what can depress the immune system. As a part of our education series, we teach about nutrition. We give hands-on cooking classes because whole food plant-based nutrition is the foundation of our treatment.

**We don't just infuse medications,
we infuse powerful information key to healing.**

Emotional healing is one of our priorities. We facilitate group sessions every week as a part of our emotional support program. Individual counseling is available too. Spiritual fortitude is key in the fight against cancer. Daily devotions,

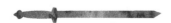

including praise and worship music, prayer and share time are a part of our spiritual care.

Oasis of Hope educates its patients about treatments, to convert them from patients to a self-healing advocates. Being a self-healing advocate is a much stronger position than being a patient that passively receives treatment. A self-healing advocate actively participates in treatment decisions and self-care.

We empower people for self-care.

CONCLUSION

As we have explained, our plan of attack includes tactics and interventions for the short-term, mid-term and long-term. In the short-term, we eliminate acute problems that pose imminent threats. If we need surgery, radiation or low dose chemotherapy, we will propose it to a patient. We explain how these interventions could buy time for our natural therapies to kick in. Our mid-term plan of attack is to educate and empower our patients to become self-healing advocates.

They can participate in getting well rather than merely receiving care from doctors in a passive manner. Also, while being treated at the hospital, we begin the long-term strategy that revolves around lifestyle medicine. As mentioned above, at the heart of this is cooking. Our incredible health coaches and cooking team-teach food preparation in a way that makes it fun, delicious and easy. You have to see our amazing teaching bar and nutrition center. We invite all of our patients to download our free mobile app, *Healthy Long Life*, which is full of recipes and demonstration videos. We even offer a bit of training in the garden to inspire our patients to grow food at home. So in the long-term, we empower everyone for self-care and encourage patients to share what they learn with their families. Education is important because a patient needs to understand what they are going to do when they go home. It is part the foundation of our comprehensive home therapy. If a patient is informed and understands why the treatment elements are essential, the better the treatment adherence is bound to be. We love empowering our patients through education. The more a patient complies with treatment, the better the result.

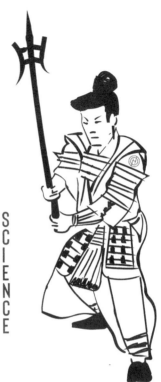

THE ART 艺术 AND

SCIENCE

科学

OF UNDERMINING 削弱

CANCER

癌

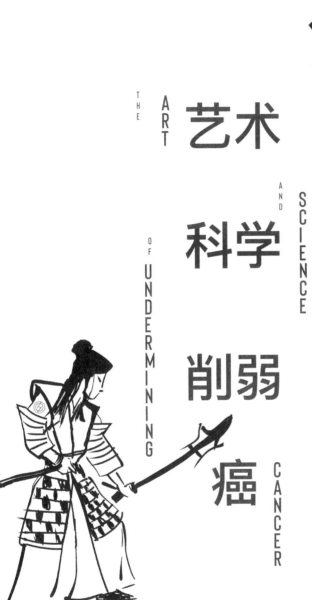

STORY OF HOPE

Steve Johnson • Hodgkin's Lymphoma • 2017

I had been sick for several years. It seemed no one could diagnose my problem. I actually went to one of the most prestigious hospitals in the country. They missed it. Then I found it, a lump on my side. What is that? The biopsy results were that it was Hodgkin's Lymphoma. How could this be? I had tried to eat healthily and be healthy.

I told my doctor, when she made the diagnosis, that I would be going to Mexico. She said, "I know, let me know if I can do anything to help." (She is an exceptional physician.) Mexico? Let me explain. There's a hospital in Tijuana called "Oasis of Hope." I knew of its treatment and results because I served as a missionary chaplain from the years 2000 to 2006. I am the man who knew too much when it comes to cancer treatment. So, I caught the next plane to San Diego.

The treatments prescribed by the Oasis of Hope doctors were not extremely invasive. Dr. Contreras did recommend chemotherapy because Hodgkin's Lymphoma responds well to conventional therapy supported by alternatives, and the cancer was in an advanced stage. He said this combination therapy had a ninety percent cure rate. The chemo was not exactly the most pleasant part of my treatment. But in the long run, it was well worth it.

My diagnosis was in April, and by August, I was nearly cancer-free. There were still a few spots to contend with, but I was in total remission after one year. I've been in total remission now for nearly three years. No question about it, Oasis of Hope is the only place to go if you have cancer.

—Steve Johnson
Weyerhaeuser, Wisconsin
USA

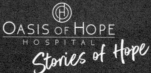

謀攻

FIVE

STRATEGIZE

Supreme excellence consists in breaking the enemy's resistance without fighting.

—Sun Tzu
The Art of War
Attack by Stratagem

On October 30, 1974, sixty thousand spectators gathered in Kinshasa, Zaire to witness *The Rumble in the Jungle*. Don King was the mastermind promoter of this historic brawl between the defending heavyweight champion of the world, George Foreman, and the great Muhammad Ali. At that point in Ali's career, he had endured some losses and setbacks. In 1967, he refused to be drafted by the Army because he was a conscientious objector. One consequence of his decision was having the heavyweight title stripped away. In 1970, the New York Supreme Court reinstated his boxing license, and he was ready to fight again. After a quick win over Jerry Quarry, he was defeated by Smokin' Joe Frazier in 1971, and Ken Norton in 1973. In January of 1974, he started his climb to the top again by defeating Joe Frazier by decision in twelve rounds. Once again, Ali earned a shot at the title. He set out to prove that he was still the greatest fighter of all time.

Ali was ready to face Foreman. The bout began at 4:30 AM in Zaire, so the televised fight could be watched at a favorable hour in the USA. The boxer who floated like a butterfly was hoping to sting like a bee to take back the most coveted sports' title— *Heavyweight Champion of the World.* The bell rang. Within seconds, Foreman began delivering the thunderous Thor-like Mjolnir hammer blows that had taken many a skilled fighter down.

Something looked off about Ali that morning. Had his butterfly wings had been clipped? Instead of floating around his opponent and landing stinging blows, Ali was not putting up a fight. Foreman unleashed a flurry of punches round after round. Ali put his arms up for protection and leaned deep back into the ropes to avoid the full force of Foreman's fury. Victory for Foreman looked certain. No one was aware that Ali was revealing a revolutionary strategy. That morning before the sun rose, the "Rope-a-Dope" strategy was born. For the first seven

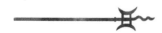

rounds, Ali didn't expend energy throwing punches or dancing around. He was the *dope* leaning on the *ropes*. By the fifth round, Foreman was visibly exhausted. In the eighth round, seemingly out of nowhere, Ali unleashed a tornado of punishing lefts and rights. The combination punches exploded out of his energy reserves. Ali hit Foreman's face, and Foreman's face hit the mat.[1] The cancer-fighting lesson here is that when facing a powerful force, a direct attack may exhaust all of your energy and resources. A *rope-a-dope* strategy can conserve needed resources for the right moment to strike.

Oasis of Hope strategies unleash combination therapies designed to kick the legs out from under cancer.

Just like Ali needed a strategy to advance against his younger and stronger opponent, it takes a comprehensive strategy to knock out cancer. This chapter will share how our strategies unleash combination therapies designed to kick the legs out from under cancer. Our master strategy is to strengthen a patient, use natural therapies to slow and reverse the progression of cancer, and teach lifestyle changes to inhibit a recurrence of cancer.

This chapter will cover why chemotherapy and radiation fail when it comes to maintaining the patient's quality of life and preventing recurrence. You will see that treatment shortcomings are often more about **how** a therapy is used than **what** is used.

In the same way Ali didn't try to take down Foremen in the first round, our approach doesn't try to take down cancer with the first round of chemotherapy. Instead, we employ therapies to build up our patients' immune systems and overall health, while steadily debilitating cancer.

DIVIDE & CONQUER

Ancient war stratagem have inspired some of our treatment tactics. We employ several of Sun Tzu's *Art of War* principles in the fight against cancer. Sun Tzu said, "He will win who knows when to fight and when not to fight."[2] We incorporate rests from cancer-attacking therapies to protect our patient's energy and immune system. During these recesses, we work on restoring a patient's health, emotional wellness and immune system so we can divide and conquer cancer. Sun Tzu said that when facing a powerful large army, it is recommended to divide the army in two and engage in two smaller battles, instead of taking on the entire united army. We follow that strategy and split the fight

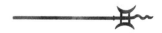

against cancer into several fronts using multiple interventions and therapies. Fighting several smaller battles is more viable than hitting cancer head on. Undermining cancer is all about dividing and conquer.

WHAT REALLY WORKS?

The main reason that alternative cancer treatment has been criticized and rejected is that it is doesn't conform to the standard research model required for FDA approval. The FDA's primary goal of the new drug approval process is to prove safety and efficacy. The drug trials must demonstrate that the benefits of a medicine outweigh the risks and adverse side effects associated with it.[3] The weakness of the FDA's criteria for drug approval is its reductionist approach. Researchers are required to isolate the active cancer-fighting agent. In clinical trials, researchers must prove what therapeutic agent works and how it works. The mode of action must be identified, along with the required dose that is safe and effective.

Alternative cancer treatments are **wholistic** versus reductionistic. Here we are using the variant spelling of "holistic" to emphasize that our treatment protocols work as a synergistic **whole**. Alternative cancer practitioners using combination therapies are wide open for criticism because there is no isolated anti-tumor agent. Imagine that an FDA evaluator visited Oasis of Hope, and this conversation took place:

FDA EVALUATOR

Please identify the active agent that is
the one that destroys cancer. Is it
A) **Amygdalin**
B) **B17**, or
C) **C** vitamin in high dose infusions?

Oasis of Hope Doctor

The answer is
D) All of the above.

Some conventional oncologists don't appreciate our synergistic strategy. They want us to demonstrate the specific drug that we use that is effective. When we reply that it isn't one drug, but it is the combination of our therapies that is working, they rebuff our work thinking it is non-scientific. In reality, all of the treatments we employ are evidence-based. Numerous clinical studies in the top peer-reviewed medical journals, in the USA and abroad, demonstrate the anticancer qualities of the therapies we prescribe. Throughout this book, we provide references to these studies for your further review. Each of our therapies provides documented benefits when used alone. But stand-alone drugs are rarely sufficient for long term victory against cancer. A combination therapy strategy is much

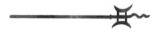

more effective. Historically, combination therapies have not been embraced by researchers and regulators because they are looking for a solo active therapeutic agent. They are in search of the mythical magic bullet.

In 2012, we sent out a scientific paper detailing the clinical trial we conducted with patients diagnosed with several different stage IV cancers. Our multi-pronged approach helped many of our patients obtain excellent results. We sent the article to a few peer-reviewed medical journals. We were pleasantly surprised at the interest that two of the top journals expressed in our study. The reviewers were impressed by our study's design, administration and results. Peer-reviewed medical journals require the identification of the sample size, structure, method, references, results, analysis, conclusion and recommendations for further studies. Our study met all of the rigorous criteria for publication. We were elated with the prospect of publication. There was just one question the reviewers from both journals asked, "In your protocol, you administered seven different therapies. Which one produced the results you achieved?" We replied and explained that it was the combination that worked. Our study did not attribute the incredible results to one specific treatment element. In reality, for one patient, one of the seven therapies may have worked. For others, multiple therapies in the combination may have been more effective. It is impossible to isolate a single treatment that works best for everyone. We know that multiple therapies given in combination render better results than treatments tested independently. "Well, doctor, if that is the case, we can't publish the report." We were temporarily deflated until *The Townsend Letter for Physicians* published our clinical study in September 2012.

DOUBLE STANDARDS

There are double standards in how medical journals apply rules to alternative cancer treatment. Most of the protocols used in cancer these days consist of combination chemotherapies like FOLFOX. The information that the National Cancer Institute provides on FOLFOX, a combination of chemotherapies approved by the FDA to treat colorectal cancer, begins with the statement:

"Chemotherapy is often given as a combination of drugs. **Combinations usually work better than single drugs because different drugs kill cancer cells in different ways.**"[4]

Wait what? Read that again, please. We put the key sentence in bold to make it easy for you to see the point we are making. If the medical journals had applied the same criteria to our

Townsend Letter: https://www.townsendletter.com/AugSept2012/metastatic0812.html

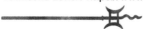

combination of therapies, as they do for combination chemotherapies, our article would have been published earlier. Let us take the liberty of writing a statement that the National Cancer Institute should publish about Oasis of Hope therapies. We will change only a few words from the NCI statement on FOLFOX:

"Oasis of Hope Alternative Cancer Treatment is often given as a combination of natural therapies, whole food plant-based nutrition and drugs. Combinations usually work better than single drugs because different therapies kill cancer cells in different ways."

Again, the trend in chemotherapy is to use combinations. Even the name FOLFOX is a combination of chemotherapies:

FOL = Leucovorin Calcium

F = Fluorouracil (5FU)

OX = Oxaliplatin

FOLFOX is made up of two chemotherapies—5FU and the aggressive oxaliplatin—and folic acid. Leucovorin calcium is a folic acid supplement that protects against the depletion of folic acid and anemia that the two chemotherapies can cause. The FDA approves combination therapies like FOLFOX, when each medication is approved before use in combination. That argument could be made for many alternative cancer treatments as well.

Today, most conventional oncology treatments involve multiple drugs. Oncologists don't know which specific drug is the one that is working or, in many cases, not working. For whatever reason, peer-reviewed journals publish results for combination chemotherapies but have traditionally rejected combination natural therapies. It is hypocritical.

Oasis of Hope *Core* and *Enhanced* protocols weaken cancer, target and kill cancerous cells, and restore the immune system.

MULTIPRONGED APPROACH

Our fifty-seven plus years of experience form the foundation of our protocols for strategic advancement against cancer. Our strategy is a multi-pronged approach to slow, control or reverse cancer. We look at cancer as a chronic disease to be managed. Oasis of Hope *Core* and *Enhanced* protocols employ various therapies. Each treatment has individual therapeutic objectives. Some of our treatments weaken cancer, some target and kill cancer cells, and others restore the patient's immune system. Our treatment also includes emotional and spiritual support. Our strategy is rather complex, but if you look at the whole picture, it makes practical and scientific sense. A strategic, holistic advance against cancer, that employs combination therapies, is why so many of our patients enjoy

better results than others being treated at conventional oncology centers.

Oasis of Hope therapies address chemoresistance and fight against cancer recurrence.

CHEMOTHERAPY CYCLES CAN BE VICIOUS CYCLES

It is imperative to address the issues of chemo-resistance and recurrence. It is common for chemotherapy to have a good initial response. A patient may think he is out of the woods, but in follow up visits, his doctor reveals test results indicating that cancer has come back. Additional cycles of chemotherapy are given in hopes that it will work the way it did in the first round. Often, the tumor doesn't respond as well because it has developed resistance to the chemotherapy used initially. The next step is to use more aggressive second-line chemotherapies that may lead to another partial remission. It is a vicious cycle of destroying cancer, recurrence and then using more aggressive chemotherapies. The cycle stops when the patient can no longer tolerate treatment. Usually the patient's cancer evolves to stage IV by the time chemo options are exhausted.

A cold way to look at the conventional oncology strategy is that increasingly potent and aggressive chemotherapies are given until the cancer is destroyed, or the patient cannot tolerate treatment and is put on hospice. Conventional therapies are extremely toxic, and patients have to stop treatment with them at some point. Alternative therapies are non-toxic and can be given as long as needed.

In a cancer fight, you can never drop your guard.

DON'T DROP YOUR GUARD

The problem with discontinuing treatment is that the recurrence rate of advanced-stage cancer is very high. Stopping treatment is like dropping your guard, which results in cancer coming back with a vengeance. As mentioned above, cancer often comes back resistant to treatment. There is also an emotional component. Cancer inspires fear, and when it goes into remission, the emotional relief can result in a person dropping their guard. It's understandable. When an oncologist tells a patient that treatment was successful, and there is no sign of active cancer, the patient breathes a huge sigh of relief. Few patients have the understanding that a recurrence may be waiting just around the corner. In a cancer fight, you can never afford to drop your guard. Even when Mohammad Ali was on the ropes, he never dropped his guard. He had respect for the power of Foreman's punches, and their potential to take him down.

Oncologists understand the potential for cancer to come back and take the patient down. But they prescribe additional treatments that may take the patient down quicker than the disease. Even in a moment of partial remission, oncologists are aware that results will not be lasting and often recommend more chemotherapy or radiation as a preventive measure. The patient may be confused and question the doctor saying, "There is no disease, why do you want to put me through such aggressive therapy?" The answer is that conventional therapy has no other strategy other than an aggressive direct attack on cancer. So even when a patient could do better without additional harmful doses of chemotherapy or radiation, the threat of recurrence is significant and oncologists will strongly recommend additional treatment. When a patient understands the reality of the vicious chemotherapy cycle, they may live in fear even when a partial remission is achieved.

THE PROBLEM WITH THE CONVENTIONAL ONCOLOGY STRATEGY

Chemotherapy, radiation and surgery depress the immune system. This conventional oncology problem is perilous because a patient's immune system must be functioning optimally for long-lasting results to be achieved. Using increasingly aggressive chemotherapies, or radiation when there is a recurrence of cancer, is like a person who lives in a high-crime neighborhood where someone throws a rock through one of the windows of his house. To prevent another crime, he has the police come and aggressively break the rest of his windows so criminals won't. He hasn't prevented anything. He has further damaged his home and left it wide open for burglars to walk right in. That is pretty much how immune-depressing chemotherapy and radiation work. It isn't logical because the only thing that can prevent recurrence is a fully functioning immune system.

Oasis of Hope protocols rebuild and fortify our patients' immune systems.

In the above example of the high crime neighborhood, the home is the body, and the windows represent the immune system. The windows are in place to keep the criminals out, or expel them from the house. The criminals are mutated cells that want to invade the house, reproduce and eventually fill the house. The police represent conventional oncology therapies.

Mutated cells may break a window, but the logical response isn't to have the police break all the windows. Destroying more windows will further expose the home to additional invaders. Instead, the homeowner should call in a construction team to rebuild the window and fortify the other windows so that they won't be broken. Conventional therapy is void of a strategy like a construction team that rebuilds and fortifies the body and its immune system.

HOW TO ACHIEVE LONG-LASTING RESULTS

We are people of faith. We believe that all healing comes through and by the *Great Physician*. It concerns us, however, when we see a church member undergo chemotherapy, go into remission, and then get up in front of their congregation to testify about a miraculous healing. It feels like the other shoe could drop at any time. Sadly, if a patient only has conventional therapy, the likelihood of a cancer recurrence is high because it is debilitating. It destroys a patient's immune system, and has no plan for staving off a recurrence. Cancer remission followed by a recurrence is like an army that wins a battle, but not the war. It takes some territory for a short time only because the enemy will regroup and take the land back. Even when cancer is toppled, a recurrence is always possible. When a person receives a miracle, preventive measures are still necessary. Let us reiterate that we don't deny that Jesus heals.

Our core belief is that all healing comes from Jesus Christ.

But here is a key question: **How do you maintain your miracle?** You could rephrase the question to be: **How can long-lasting results be achieved?** Addressing this question is crucial because the recurrence rates of various types of cancer can be quite high.

The recurrence rate for each type of cancer varies. For instance, statistics indicate that forty percent of women who have had breast cancer will experience a recurrence during their lifetimes.[5] Cancer of the pancreas has a recurrence rate of seventy-four percent.[6] For lung cancer, the recurrence rate is seventy-five percent.[7] Fighting against cancer recurrence is an imperative strategic tactic we employ. That is where the Oasis of Hope strategy shines and can often improve the quality of life of a patient and help them live far beyond his original prognosis.

When a patient experiences excellent results and the prognosis looks good for the long-term, we change tactics. We don't prescribe aggressive therapies to continue a direct assault

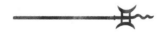

on cancer. Instead, we ask the patient to work with us to consolidate the results and prevent a recurrence by building up the immune system. Promoting natural defenses is essential because most of our patients come to us with late-stage cancers, and have experienced multiple recurrences. Most have endured chemotherapy or radiation, and favorable results did not last long.

Oasis of Hope protocols often improve the quality of life, and help people live far beyond the original prognosis.

Our strategic advancement goes beyond the initial battle. We build up defenses because we know the enemy will regroup and try to attack again. It is a given, and so we address it. Conventional oncology uses short-term strategies focused on destroying the initial threat posed by cancer. Oasis of Hope uses a long-term strategy. Conventional therapies sometimes cure stage I or stage II cancers. But conventional therapies' success rates are not good for advanced stage metastatic cancer. Traditional oncology treatments are so toxic they cannot be given indefinitely. We design therapies with natural elements that can be used for a long time, years if necessary.

A LONG-TERM HEALTHY MENTALITY

At Oasis of Hope, we partner with our patients for the long run. We include follow up consultations for five years at no charge because we know that we need to help our patients overcome the fear of recurrence. The power of the mind is incredibly strong. In our strategy, we support patients over the long term emotionally as well. We help patients adopt a positive mentality about the lifestyle changes they will need to make. A change in mindset can be as powerful, or more powerful than the medications we give. When we help our patients understand the value of their lives, they become motivated to fight to survive and protect all of the favorable results they achieve.

Your mindset is as powerful as our medicine.

MIRACLE STEWARDSHIP

We consider all positive outcome results from our treatment protocols miracles, or a gift if you will. Miracles need to be responsibly maintained. We encourage our patients to be good stewards of their miracles. It is not valid to think, "Well, I made it, I did it," and then go back to old bad habits of the lifestyle that triggered cancer in the first place. That is a sure

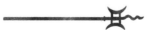

recipe for a recurrence. We help people develop a mentality that embraces lifestyle changes that can build the immune system and maintain the achieved healing. You will have to make sacrifices and make some changes if you want long-term results.

Consider people that have gastric bypass surgery. This type of surgery is incredibly effective and often results in patients losing one hundred pounds or more. But, if a patient does not adopt new healthy eating habits, over a period of three to four years, they will gain much of the weight back and get on track to regain all of the weight over time. Surgically induced weight loss without making a lifestyle change will only produce short-term success.

Lots of people want to beat cancer without making a lifestyle change. But every goal in life requires preparation, sacrifice and change. Your health goals are no exception. Health is a gift that we generally don't appreciate until we lose it. If you knock cancer down, you must make lifestyle changes so that cancer will not rise again.

IT'S A SPRINT & A MARATHON

We don't understand why conventional oncologists look down on alternative, natural, and integrative therapies, without even reading the supporting scientific evidence. Equally as dumbfounding are natural health practitioners that repudiate any use of conventional medication because of possible adverse side effects. When talking about surgery, radiation and chemotherapy, they often use very aggressive terminology such as slash, burn and poison. At Oasis of Hope, we don't strictly fall into either the conventional or the alternative medicine camp. We fall into the patient's camp. To keep cancer off balance, we may modulate between alternative treatments and conventional therapies.

Oasis of Hope practices patient-focused, data-driven medicine.

The Oasis of Hope brand of medicine is one that seeks to extend life, minimize side effects, rebuild the immune system and improve our patients' quality of life. We practice patient-focused, data-driven medicine. Oasis of Hope's integrative cancer treatment gives patients every advantage against cancer, whether it is a pharmaceutical or a natural element.

For long-term success, we try to meet the individual needs of each patient. We don't use terms like slash, burn and poison.

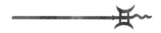

We employ therapies that provide the best benefits without taking an unnecessary toll on our patient's quality of life.

Cancer is both a sprint and a marathon. The sprint aspect of cancer is that sometimes an acute condition, like a blocked colon, will require a conventional intervention to buy time for the patient to respond to natural therapies. The marathon aspect of cancer is that lifestyle changes are necessary for the rest of a person's life.

To clarify, we may employ conventional therapies to resolve a life-threatening situation and buy time for natural therapies to kick in. Do you remember what we tell people who criticize our use of conventional treatments? We tell them that we practice good medicine, not conventional or alternative medicine. In our experience, a strategy that integrates both conventional and alternative treatments gets the best results.

Circling back around, chemotherapy alone is useful in very few types of cancer, such as childhood leukemia and lymphomas. In early-stage operable cancers, surgery can often be curative. For stage IV cancers, we must go beyond chemotherapy, radiation and surgery. We need to employ alternative treatments that can keep cancer off balance and be used for the long haul.

HOW LONG DOES TREATMENT LAST?

Some people expect that one visit to Oasis of Hope will get rid of cancer. Remember, cancer is a marathon, not just a sprint. The number and frequency of visits to our hospital depend on a patient's evolving condition. We recommend patients with a twenty percent to thirty percent tumor activity reduction to return to us for boosters every three months. We can stretch out the time between treatments to six months or more for patients that experience a reduction in tumor activity by seventy percent to eighty percent. The number of visits to our hospital depends on variables such as how aggressive a tumor is, the quantity and types of therapies required, and the patient's prognosis.

CONCLUSION

We would like to end this chapter with a miracle case that continues to play out in the life of one of our lovely patients named Natalie. We cannot say that her results are typical. Treatment outcomes vary from patient to patient. What we can say, is that most of our patients will have some benefits, and in a relatively high number of cases, a prolonged remission is achieved. Let's get into Natalie's story.

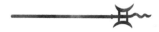

A WONDERFUL SUCCESS STORY: NATALIE MERFALEN

Here is a great story of where our one-two-three-punch has been effective. We received Natalie five years ago. She had been diagnosed with very aggressive thyroid cancer. Her initial response to conventional treatment was favorable. She had surgery to remove the tumor. Then she received radiation therapy, which obtained a partial remission for a year. As happens in so many cases, the tumor came back, and conventional therapy was no longer a favorable option. The standard treatment plan was failing.

Natalie was young, single and had no children. But, she had a vision of beating cancer and starting a family. With this motivation, she decided to come to us for an alternative to chemotherapy, radiation and surgery. She started our treatment protocol, leveraging the one-two-three punch strategy. Her treatment commenced with three weeks of oxidative therapy at the hospital. Then, she began our anti-oxidative home therapy for three months. The tumor in her throat diminished by more than fifty percent. We continued treating her and keeping cancer off balance. After a year, a PET scan confirmed that she was totally disease-free. She now comes to the hospital about every nine months for re-evaluation. She has been responsible with her healing and has made the lifestyle changes necessary for long-term success. Not only has she beaten cancer, but she has also realized her dream. She is now married and is the proud mother of a beautiful baby girl!

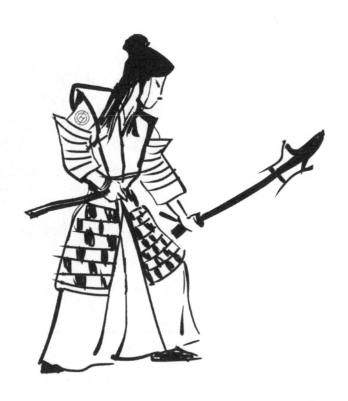

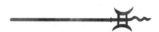

STORY OF HOPE

Michelle Frisch • Stage II Breast Cancer HR+- • 2016

June 2016 was the first time I even suspected something was wrong. I felt a lump in my breast first, and then in my throat. Though I thought it could never happen to me, somewhere deep inside me, I already knew the test result would be positive. I loved Jesus. I was living overseas doing missions work for crying out loud! Yet, here I was, sitting in the doctor's office full of shock and fear. I was diagnosed with stage two breast cancer HR+. The good news was that this was the most common kind. The bad news, it was aggressive. If I tried to do anything but chemo, it was suicide.

I had just turned 40, my oldest daughter was about to start her senior year of high school, my boys were going into 10th and 5th grades, and my baby girl was going into 4th grade. This can't be real! The fear was overwhelming. I had always been a person of faith. I clung to Jesus in the darkness. My husband was so supportive, but what could he do? I felt alone in this diagnosis. The only thing I knew could make a real difference—my only chance at living—was Jesus. Did I really think he could heal me? Did I think I was worth healing? I struggled with this concept and couldn't sleep for countless nights. I was so afraid that I needed to be with someone all the time, so I followed my husband to our church.

One night I was wrestling with this, so I laid on the floor and begged God to heal me. I praised Him for making our bodies with such vast complexity and gave my body back to him figuratively. I wasn't worry-free from that moment on, but I did see God's reminders to me everywhere I looked. The song "Diamonds" came out on the radio around that time, and I loved it and sang it wholeheartedly! I started seeing diamonds everywhere. I saw them on signs, and friends would send me them in the mail. It was as if Jesus was saying to me I am with YOU in this...here is a reminder!!

In the first few months, my doctor wanted to do lots of tests. I had no previous knowledge of anything regarding cancer, as I was the first one in my family to be diagnosed. I read everything I could get my hands on, and one of the books I checked out from the library was Dr. Contreras' book *Beating Cancer: 20 Natural, Spiritual, & Medical Remedies.* All the testing took time, which suited me just fine as I was on my own mission to learn how to put myself in the best position to heal. I began juicing carrots and basically lived on them and salads with no dressing. I was eating raw broccoli before my carrot juice breakfast and all kinds of crazy extreme things. I drank thirty-six ounces of carrot juice a day. I had green powder in between and a huge salad for dinner. Every day. No cheating. I went from eating McDonalds to this regimen overnight. I know you think you HAVE to have meat, but when I thought about being alive for my kids, I had to do everything I could to get to that goal. Not even a steak was going to keep me from that! I lost about thirty-five pounds and people looked at me and talked to me as if I was dying because I was so thin. I felt great though, like I was a kid again and could climb a tree with the slightest of ease!

I did this for four months until test results came back. My tumor had gotten slightly larger. I realized it may have been swollen from being under attack, or may have just been misdiagnosed the first time around. I couldn't believe that after all I had done that it was not substantially smaller! I was horrified! I was afraid that it wasn't enough and wondered what else could I do? We decided to do the unthinkable and go over the Mexican border to get help. Everything I read about Oasis of Hope was exactly what I wanted, and my non-alternative medicine husband loved that they had chemotherapy there if I needed it! People thought we were crazy. No one we knew had ever done this. Just follow the doctor's orders seemed to be the prevailing thought. But I had to do what I believed would keep me with my family. From the moment we got in the Oasis of Hope van I felt at peace. They shuttled us over the border and we went into what seemed like a hotel with a private room. For the first time since hearing that dreaded word, I felt I had a whole team of people who were really invested in ME personally. I wasn't treated just like another patient in a long list of patients. I knew everyone there had a story like mine. The meals were like round table therapy as we shared our stories. The friends I have made are my friends for life, and yes, I have had to say goodbye to some of them, but there are so many that are still here living their life that I can only say, "Glory to God and thank God for Oasis of Hope!"

One of the things that stand out as amazing at Oasis of Hope is the food they prepare and serve is TOP NOTCH. If you're coming from the SAD (Standard American Diet), it will be shocking. But knowing EVERYTHING you see is safe to eat is an amazing relief!!! Also, you can receive your IV treatment in a community room as an option. I often had mine while listening to the pastor lead live worship music. It's a fantastic way to receive care for your body, mind and spirit simultaneously. They also offer cooking classes so you can make some of their amazing foods back at home. The breathing and walking classes were also really fun. I was able to relax, get solid answers to all of my questions, and get some really cool, specialized treatments while being monitored. I know God brought me to Oasis of Hope, and I can't say enough good things about it. If you are on the fence, what do you really have to lose!!!!!! Oh, by the way, in April 2017, I had my first CLEAN SCAN report!

—Michelle Frisch
Fall River, Massachusetts
USA

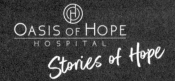

軍形

SIX

DEFEND

The good fighters of old put themselves beyond the possibility of defeat, and then wait for an opportunity of defeating the enemy.

—Sun Tzu
The Art of War
Tactical Dispositions

Leonardo • Raphael • Michelangelo • Donatello. Do you know who these guys are? If you think they are the most prominent and influential artists of the Renaissance era, you would not be incorrect. But, we are talking about the more famous namesakes, you know, the ones who have saved the world from mutants, aliens and the super-villain *The Shredder*. Yes, you guessed it—

T M N T

Teenage Mutant Ninja Turtles

These lovable exoskeleton youth may be the ultimate superheroes because they have built-in body armor. How cool is that? In contrast, Batman and Ironman rely on specialized high tech suits to protect them from their foes. The TMNTs were birthed in 1983 by the creative team of Peter Laird and Kevin Eastman. Their shells have stood the test of time, and they are in that legendary category of famous personalities who are enjoyed by their original fans, and the children of their fans.[1]

Much like real turtles, TMNTs have been saved by their shells countless times. A real turtle's key to survival is not a great offense; it is a great defense. The shell protects turtles from predators that may attack from any direction. Nutrition is foundational in developing a turtle's protection. Turtles love to chomp down on crustaceans, a rich source of the calcium needed to build and maintain a hard healthy shell.[2]

Nutrition is essential for developing the best defense against cancer—your immune system.

Why all the turtle talk? Well, you have something in common with them. Nutrition is essential for developing your best defense against cancer—your immune system. A study published in 2018 on micronutrients and immune function stated, "The first line of defense is innate immunity."[3] The article outlines the need for specific micronutrients needed to bolster the immune system. The article specifies, "Various micronutrients are essential for immune-competence, particularly vitamins A, C, D, E, B2, B6, and B12, folic acid, iron, selenium, and zinc."[3]

At Oasis of Hope, we embrace and maximize the cancer-fighting potential derived from a designer nutrition program. We incorporate foods rich in anticancer nutrients that can turn oncogenes off, food that is low on the glycemic index to avoid feeding the cancer cells by the rapid conversion of food into glucose in the bloodstream, and foods that are high in fiber and low in animal protein and fat. Building a good defense starts

with getting the right information. The first thing that comes to mind about getting informed is the common proverb, "Practice makes perfect," because that's not necessarily true. If you practice wrong, you will never become perfect. So it's perfect practice that makes perfect. As far as information is concerned, accurate information will be very good for you and misinformation can be devastating. It is crucial to discern between accurate and false information.

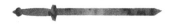

Louis Pasteur said, "Chance favors only the prepared mind." Pasteur's statement is poignant if your plan of achievement is to leave things to chance. His astute observation teaches that you must prepare if chance is to favor you. Consider this. There are many opportunities in life that will pass you by if you're not prepared to seize them. Preparation starts with identifying available opportunities and resources. Get informed, so opportunities don't pass you by. Our principal motivation for writing this book is to empower you with accurate information and prepare you for healing opportunities. Evidence-based information is paramount in your fight against cancer. Before we dig into the main theme of this chapter, which how nutrition affects cancer, allow us to touch on a few other important topics.

HOW TO TALK ABOUT CANCER

It isn't easy to break the news of a cancer diagnosis with family and friends. Sharing such news, in a sense, makes it real. Being in denial is no longer an option. We see this with many patients. It is challenging to disclose the distressing situation while keeping positive. Family members may enter denial in a fear response. If you are the one with cancer, you can be an ambassador and teach your family whatever you learn about effective cancer treatment and prevention. We encourage you to seize this great opportunity. By teaching your family what you learn on your cancer journey, you can help them reduce the risk of developing cancer.

A benefit for your family can rise out of your health crises. Did you know you can impact your family's health and epigenetic information that is passed on? Changes in nutrition and lifestyle can modify the gene expression of inherited genes. So even if there are cancer-associated genes in the family, they can be overcome. Changes in diet and exercise are the two factors that have the greatest potential for helping your loved ones prevent cancer.

Many people are resistant to a message of change in lifestyle. But, when a family member gets cancer, people pay attention. Capture this mega wake-up call for the benefit of your family. You are an inspiration to your loved ones. You can advise them on how to adopt lifestyle changes that reduce their risk of developing cancer.

A WORLD WITHOUT CANCER

A world without cancer starts with preventive measures. I learned a fascinating concept, on a recent trip to the Max Planck Institute's Department of Aging, talking to one of its

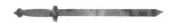

researchers who shared the correlation they found between Insulin-Like Growth Factor (IGF-1) and aging.[5] It is relevant to cancer treatment and prevention because a diet that promotes the overproduction of IGF-1 is deleterious to our health. IGF-1 and IGF-2 can be beneficial for malignant cells because they can provoke a cascade of cell signaling transduction that is central to processes involved in oncogenesis.[6]

Many studies indicate that controlling IGF is necessary for longevity. The key to not overproducing IGF and prolonging your life is eating less animal protein and animal fat. Caloric restriction is the only action that all researchers agree on when it comes to longevity. The less you eat, the less IGF is produced. For our patients, we don't decrease calories; we change out the foods that promote IGF production for foods that control it.

Cancer thrives on sugar.

GLYCEMIC INDEX

One fact we have stressed is that cancer thrives on sugar (glucose). Cutting out candy, cakes and ice cream is a step in the right direction. But, most people are entirely unaware that all food is converted into glucose. The speed at which food is converted determines how available it is to cancer cells. There is an index that gives all foods a rating from 0 to 100, with pure sugar (glucose) being 100. It's called the *Glycemic Index* (GI). Harvard Medical School explains what GI is well, stating, "The lower a food's glycemic index, the slower blood sugar rises after eating that food. In general, the more cooked or processed a food is, the higher its GI, and the more fiber or fat in a food, the lower its GI."[7]

The National Cancer Institute defines GI as:

A measure of the increase in the level of blood glucose (a type of sugar) caused by eating a specific carbohydrate (food that contains sugar) compared with eating a standard amount of glucose. Foods with a high glycemic index release glucose quickly and cause a rapid rise in blood glucose. Foods with a low glycemic index release glucose slowly into the blood. A relationship between the glycemic index and recurrent colorectal cancer is being studied.[8]

Did you notice that even the National Cancer Institute is studying the relationship between high GI foods and recurrent colorectal cancer? There is a relationship between high GI foods and all cancer, because tumors grow faster when glucose is easily accessed. As an introduction to Oasis of Hope's nutrition program, consider the critical observation made in the above Harvard Medical School statement:

The more cooked or processed a food is, the higher its GI, and the more fiber or fat in a food, the lower its GI.[7]

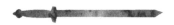

At Oasis of Hope, we have developed a nutrition program that has a moderate amount of cooked foods, no processed foods, plenty of high-fiber foods and a portion of healthy fats. Let's get into how we use food to build your turtle shell (immune system) protection as an added way to defend against cancer progression. This information is also something you can pass on to your family to help them defend themselves against cancer.

When fighting cancer, sometimes the best offense is a great defense.

QUASI-VEGAN DIETS LOWER CANCER RATES

Oasis of Hope recommends that its patients consume a predominantly whole food plant-based diet. We provide modest amounts of high quality protein serving small portions of fish and eggs to patients to avoid muscle mass loss. Our recommendation is based on countless studies and reports from around the world.

The age-adjusted death rates for several cancers prominent in western countries are five-fold to ten-fold lower in cultures whose traditional diets are primarily based on whole plant-based foods. Cancers of the breast, prostate, colorectal, pancreatic, ovarian, and leukemia are very common and in Western cultures. Hence, they are occasionally referred to as Western cancers. The incidence rates for these types of cancer are lower in countries whose diets have modest protein content relative to diets found in more affluent societies.[9,10] Such diets are sometimes referred to as "quasi-vegan." "Age-adjusted" refers to the risk of dying of cancer at any given age. In other words, lower cancer mortality in these societies is not because people are unlikely to attain the advanced ages when cancer is more prevalent. Indeed, once people in these societies survive the rigors of infancy and childhood, they have an excellent chance to achieve the same lifespan that we do.

Not all cancers are low in these societies. Cancers of the liver, stomach and esophagus are relatively common. In these countries, poor hygiene—not the diet—exposes populations to infectious agents or carcinogens that cause these specific cancers.

Several factors may contribute to the decidedly lower cancer rates associated with quasi-vegan diets. Whole food plant-based diets are rich in phytochemicals that help detoxify carcinogens and DNA damaging free radicals.[11,12] Plant-based nutrition is void of heme iron, an organic form of iron found in flesh foods, especially red meat. Heme iron is efficiently absorbed even when the body already has ample iron stores.[13] High body iron levels may increase the risk of mutagenic damage to DNA.[14,15] The body iron stores of vegans and vegetarians tend to be about half as high as those of omnivores.[16] Cooking meat at high heat produces cancer-causing chemicals called heterocyclic amines. That is not the case in plant foods cooked at comparable heat. The compound creatine is found only in flesh foods, is an essential precursor for heterocyclic amine production.[17,18]

PLANT-BASED DIETS DECREASE IGF-I ACTIVITY

Let's circle back to insulin-like growth factor-I (IGF-I), specifically the relationship between high IGF-I levels and cancer promotion. Moderate-protein vegan diets lower the liver's production IGF-I, which helps control cancer. IGF-I has often been referred to as a "universal cancer promoter."[19] A high proportion of the body's cells are responsive to this growth factor, as they carry IGF-I receptors. IGF-I acts on tissues to accelerate the multiplication of cells. At the same time, it tends to block a protective process known as "apoptosis."[11] Apoptosis is a type of cell suicide that is evoked when a cell "senses" that its DNA has sustained damage too extensive to repair. It is crucial to eliminate cells that have damaged DNA. Some types of mutagenic damage to DNA can affect a cell's growth control mechanisms, such that it becomes more likely to reproduce without restraint—a characteristic of pre-cancerous cells as well as cancers. When IGF-I activity suppresses apoptosis, mutated cells' survival may increase, and they could acquire more mutations. Full-fledged cancer could arise as a result. The dual effect of IGF-I on cellular proliferation and apoptosis can increase the rate at which cells acquire mutations, while blunting the self-protective mechanisms that eliminate such cells. Not surprisingly, epidemiological studies have found that people with relatively high IGF-I levels in their bloodstream are more prone to developing many Western cancers.[20-21] Studies in rodents show that high IGF-I levels can also drive the aggressive growth and spread of the many cancers that are responsive to this growth factor.[22,23]

HOW NUTRITION CAN SLOW CANCER'S GROWTH & SPREAD

The ability of quasi-vegan diets to lower circulating levels of IGF-I has been demonstrated both in rodent studies and in humans.[24-27] Furthermore, protein-restricted diets have been shown to lower IGF-I levels, restricting the growth of human cancers implanted in immunodeficient mice.[28] Studies at the

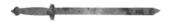

Pritikin Institute have shown that blood serum derived from patients who have adopted a quasi-vegan diet for several weeks is less able to sustain the proliferation and block apoptosis in cultured human prostate cancer cells, compared with serum derived from people eating high-protein omnivore diets.[29,30] Analogously, in a study conducted at Dr. Dean Ornish's clinic, the PSA levels of patients with early prostate cancer (before surgery, in the so-called "watchful waiting" phase) rose less quickly in patients eating a quasi-vegan whole food Pritikin diet (while also exercising, and practicing stress-control techniques), than in those eating the more typical American diet.[31,32]

IGF-I highly determines the risk of prostate cancer. Indeed, one study compared the age-adjusted death rate from prostate cancer in countries eating quasi-vegan diets (less than ten percent animal protein), with countries eating diets high in animal products. The death rate was fifteen-fold higher in omnivore countries.[10] Conversely, there are occasional reports of marked regression of pre-existing prostate cancer in patients who adopt a plant-based diet.[33]

Over the years, Oasis of Hope has deepened its commitment to educating on the power of plant-based nutrition considering how effective it is at lowering circulating IGF-I.

HOW PLANT-BASED FOODS LOWER IGF-I

How is it that moderate-protein plant-based diets lower IGF-I levels? Recent studies have provided at least a partial answer.[34] Please hang in there with us through this section because it gets pretty technical. In the human body, proteins are synthesized from twenty compounds known as amino acids. Some of these amino acids are considered "essential" because the human body is incapable of manufacturing them from other compounds. Essential amino acids must be acquired from our diet. GCN2 is activated within our cells whenever any one of the essential amino acids is in relatively short supply. It causes specific adaptations that enable cells to cope with this situation. For example, it slows the synthesis of many proteins. But activated GCN2 also boosts the production of other proteins, notably ATF4. Within the liver, ATF4 promotes the increased synthesis of an intriguing hormone known as FGF21 (fibroblast growth factor-21). FGF21 is sometimes referred to as "the longevity hormone," because mice bioengineered to express increased levels enjoy a delay in the aging process and a markedly longer mean and maximal lifespan.[36,37] FGF21 produced in the liver can act on hepatic cells to suppress IGF-I synthesis, resulting in lower blood levels of this cancer-promoting factor.[34,36] FGF21 also acts on fat cells to boost

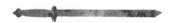

adiponectin production, which appears to have the potential to decrease the risk for certain cancers.[38-40] Adiponectin is a protein hormone produced by fat cells.

Plant-based diets tend to be lower in total protein content than animal products because they are composed primarily of protein and fat. Plant protein also tends to be lower in certain essential amino acids than animal proteins, notably the amino acids lysine and methionine.[41] A whole food plant-based diet with moderate protein content and low soy protein, or meat analogs, is decidedly lower amounts of lysine and methionine. Plant-based diets can lead to activation of GCN2 within the liver, resulting in higher production of FGF21 and lower production of IGF-I.[34] The ability of animal protein-restricted diets to slow the growth of certain human cancers in mice has been demonstrated in recent studies.[28]

Though not a cure, a whole food plant-based diet helps slow the progression of cancer.

NOT A "MAGIC BULLET"

Plant-based diets are not a magic bullet for cancer. Although it is reasonable to suspect that they will slow the growth and spread of many cancers, they rarely cause marked regression of cancers on the level of cancer treatments. Also, many cancers that were formerly responsive to IGF-I lose this sensitivity over time. They develop new mutations that can boost their growth factor signaling in the absence of IGF-I. Though not a cancer cure, a whole food plant-based diet helps slow the progression of cancer. Plant-based nutrition is the ideal foundational therapy. It works in a complementary fashion with Oasis of Hope therapies that kill or slow cancers. Moreover, whole food plant-based diets tend to be good for your health in numerous ways, including reducing risk for heart attack, stroke, diabetes, obesity and various colonic disorders.[42] These health benefits are why we employ a whole food plant-based diet of moderate protein content for our patients.

LOSS OF LEAN MUSCLE MASS PREVENTION

Cachexia is a condition that can become very serious in patients dealing with advanced-stage cancer. Cachexia is the loss of body weight, and more importantly, the loss of muscle mass.[43] When cachexia sets in, it is exceedingly difficult to reverse. It is also associated with decreased survival. For this reason, we monitor closely and take preventive measures.

Cachexia is not normal weight loss. One might assume that cancer patients lose weight because of loss of appetite due to

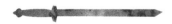

chemotherapy-provoked nausea that upsets the stomach too much to hold anything down. Though nausea is a contributing factor, cachexia involves various metabolic pathways that promote neuroendocrine hormones, pro-inflammatory cytokines and proteolysis inducing factor (PIF). Clinical studies have identified PIF as an element that provokes the loss of skeletal muscle by decreasing protein synthesis.[44]

The most important measures we can take to prevent or slow cachexia are diet and supplementation. Our nutrition program is ninety-five percent plant-based. However, due to the risk of muscle wasting our patients face, we unapologetically incorporate small amounts of fish, and occasionally eggs. Clinical data indicates that fish oil is an important protective factor against lean body mass loss. The high-quality protein in eggs may help as well.[45]

Oasis of Hope healing foods are at the heart of everything we do.

Now back to the healing power of plants. Several micronutrients are quite beneficial in the effort to keep lean muscle mass on. Curcumin, resveratrol and plant-based proteins are key.[46] To leverage plant-based nutrients, we utilize our proprietary nanoceuticals and vegan, gluten-free plant-powered protein powder.

CONCLUSION

Nutrition is one of the simplest yet elegant therapies available to your body. In the fight against cancer, defensive strategies are equally as important as offensive. Plant-based nutrition defends against inflammation-associated progression of cancer. The Oasis of Hope nutrition program is at the heart of everything we do. We use the micronutrients, present in specific foods, to starve cancer cells, inhibit the immune-suppressing inflammatory response and protect against the loss of muscle mass.

STORY OF HOPE

Nita Long • Triple-Negative Breast Cancer • 2015

When I was diagnosed with triple-negative breast cancer, it completely floored me. I had no idea that I had become a host to a ticking time bomb. After the diagnosis, the U.S. cancer system started pushing me toward their well-trodden path. We looked to our oncologist for hope, but he quickly scheduled me for a port and four months of the most aggressive chemo available before considering the removal of the tumor and undergoing radiation. Even then, the outlook held only a 34% chance of success.

Years earlier, a friend of mine had been treated by Oasis of Hope, and after talking with them, I had an alternative. When we arrived at Tijuana and stepped through the hospital doors, we knew we were in the right place. The peaceful atmosphere, attention to detail, cleanliness, smiles on the staff, and scriptures on the wall were like a gust of wind in my sails.

The strategy developed by Dr. Contreras and his team was to remove the fast-growing tumor and build my body's natural immunity while applying scientifically advanced therapies. I believed in that approach much more than the option given to me in the U.S. With a foe like triple-negative breast cancer, confidence in your treatment is a must. It felt so right to strengthen my immune system instead of killing it with chemo.

Success was quick for me with a great response from the surgery and immune therapies. After the three weeks, we returned home and continued the protocol with a close connection to the Oasis of Hope team.

Two small recurrences were taken care of right away, and for the last five years, my PET scans and blood work have reflected total remission. We are blessed to have Oasis of Hope as our alternative to chemo and radiation, which can cause many additional problems.

—Nita Long
Omaha, Nebraska
United States

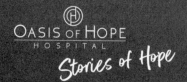

兵勢

SEVEN

ATTACK INDIRECTLY

In battle, there are two methods of attack—direct and indirect;
Yet these two in combination give rise
to an endless series of maneuvers.

—Sun Tzu
The Art of War
Energy

Shade. Did you know you can throw it? Has anyone thrown shade on you lately? If you are over the age of twenty, you may not get the question. We are well beyond that age group, so we didn't know what it meant either. Thank goodness for the *Urban Dictionary* that tells us the meaning of youthful slang.

THROW SHADE:

To say a rude or slick comment towards another person with little or no one else catching the insult except who it was directed towards.[1]

Throwing shade is a shady thing to do. It's an indirect criticism that can still really hurt. I'm convinced that kids throw shade on their parents all of the time, and thank God, we have no idea what they are talking about because we might get our feelings hurt.

When we traveled for the *Healthy Long Life* documentary series, I remember going through immigration in London and the officer asking about the purpose of my visit.

I heard one of my daughters, mind you, I'm not sure which, say, "Immigration officers must hear a lot about different movie productions." The other snickered. The comment was seemingly not directed at anybody. It didn't even use words that would signal that it was an attack. But, I picked up on the shade. I have to admit that I was pretty excited to be filming. I would enthusiastically talk about it with anyone who would listen. I had not realized that I was putting my family on pause every time I started conversations about the documentary. My daughters are sweet and patiently wait for me. But, their concern at that moment was all the jet-lagged people waiting in line behind us. They threw shade so I wouldn't slow down the immigration line by giving the unabridged answer to the simple question, "What's the purpose of your visit?"

Message received. I gave a one-word answer, "Business." The passport was stamped, and the line moved forward efficiently. I know my daughters love me and didn't intend to hurt my feelings. Still, sometimes an indirect comment makes the point without having to get into a long explanation. In cancer treatment, an indirect attack is often the most effective. The basis for this book is how to undermine cancer, not how to run it over. Undermining is an indirect attack.

INFLAMMATION IS KEY

An excellent opportunity to undermine cancer is to exploit and interfere with malignant cells' metabolic traits. Inflammation is key to cancer's promotion and growth. From their early developmental stages, all cancers thrive because of inflammation. It's essential to understand why this is so important for the tumors.

The inflammatory response is a process critical to our survival when facing acute health problems. Pathogens like bacteria and viruses can cause inflammation. It can be caused by burns, physical injuries, exposure to severe heat or cold, radiation, chemicals, allergens, toxic metals, damaged DNA, and even stress or over-excitement. Inflammation is the immune response when tissues are injured. When tissue damage occurs, a series of cell signaling induces the activation of leukocytes and directs them to the injury site. Cytokines are produced that provoke the inflammatory response.[2] Without inflammation, our bodies would be incapable of healing. That is true for acute health problems.

Just think about when you hit your thumb with a hammer or you get an infection. Your body responds protectively to repair the damage. Once the damage is repaired, the inflammation process goes away.

In the immune response, the primary defense agents in our body are the white blood cells. White blood cells are a family of many different cells. One thing that happens after a trauma, or the beginning of an infection, is that a high amount of white cells are produced and released. Our body responds to an injury or invader by producing the transcription factor nuclear factor kappa-light-chain-enhancer of activated B cells, referred to as NF Kappa B (NF-κB.)

Transcription factors are molecules that control the behavior of genes. The transcription factor NF-κB is essential for the rapid production and release of white blood cells. Typically, our white blood cell count is about 6,000, but when you have an infection, NF-κB bolsters it up to 20,000. NF-κB counteracts apoptosis, which is vital during a crisis as white

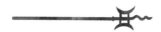

blood cells have a tremendously short life span. [3] White cells last between a few hours and a few days before they die through the apoptotic process. NF-κB anti-apoptotic action extends the white cells' lifespan. In a crisis, not only do we want those cells to be abundant so they can repair tissue damage, but we want them to be long lasting so that they can prevent any additional issues from developing, such as infection.

The inflammatory immune response ceases once the repairing process is complete. As a result, NF-κB levels reduce, overproduction stops, and the white cells die at their allotted time. That is what happens where everything is working correctly. That is the good news about NF-κB.

Here is the bad news about NF-κB. The relationship between cancer and NF-κB is mutually beneficial. NF-κB's actions of promoting cell proliferation and apoptosis shielding benefit cancer.[4]   NF-κB benefits from cancer because tumors upregulate the production of NF-κB. Tumors secrete factors that activate NF-κB, and mutated genes encode NF-κB, which causes more production.[5] When cancer cells are destroyed, the pro-inflammatory cytokine tumor necrosis factor (TNF) solicits the immune inflammatory response, which malignant cells use to proliferate.[6]

Wherever there is cancer, there is going to be a high rate of NF-κB. Researchers Aggarwal and Sung wrote, "Activation of NF-κB has been linked to various cellular processes in cancer, including inflammation, transformation, proliferation, angiogenesis, invasion, metastasis, chemoresistance, and radioresistance."[7] Notice that NF-κB even makes tumors resistant to chemotherapy and radiotherapy.

Therefore, a fundamental strategy is to diminish or neutralize NF-κB production. Several natural elements can inhibit NF-κB, such as pregnenolone and resveratrol.[8] We provide these nutrients to our patients. The problem is that the quantities needed are more than a person can ingest. It's for this reason that we employ COX-2 inhibitors to suppress the activation of NF-κB.

OFF-LABEL USE OF COX-2 INHIBITORS

Researchers have developed countless therapies to address gene mutations by upregulating or downregulating the production of specific proteins. To date, no medication has been developed specifically to downregulate the production of NF-κB. Fortunately, some medications inhibit the production of Cyclooxygenase-2 (COX-2). COX-2 is an enzyme that promotes inflammation by increasing the production of cytokines, including NF-κB. By inhibiting COX-2, NF-κB levels will also be reduced. COX-2 inhibitors were developed and approved for the treatment of arthritis. Using them as a cancer adjuvant is an off-label drug use. But, it is important to inhibit COX-2 because of its relationship with cancer. Cancer benefits from COX-2 production, and COX-2 levels are promoted by tumors. Oncogenes, growth factors, and chemotherapy increase COX-2 production. COX-2 levels are high in premalignant and malignant tissues.[9]

The best-known COX-2 inhibiting agent is aspirin, which means that aspirin has an anticancer quality. Studies indicate that low-dose aspirin can help prevent some types of cancer and inhibit metastases.[10] Aspirin may lower the risk for colorectal cancer, gastrointestinal cancer, melanoma, and ovarian, and pancreatic cancer. [11]

Unfortunately, oncologists can't tell a cancer patient, "Take two aspirin and call me in the morning," because aspirin also inhibits COX-1, a pro-coagulating agent. The amount of aspirin required to lower NF-κB sufficiently would disable a patient's blood from being able to clot. Overuse of aspirin could lead to death by gastrointestinal bleeding, so we do not include it in our protocol. Instead, our researchers identified a nonsteroidal anti-inflammatory drug (NSAID), called Celebrex, that inhibits

COX-2 but doesn't affect COX-1. Another potent COX-2 inhibitor is Dexamethasone, which is commercially called Alin.[12] We routinely prescribe Celebrex or Alin depending on how well the patient tolerates one or the other.

DOES OASIS OF HOPE USE CBD & THC?

Let's talk about cannabinoids and COX-2 inhibitors. Celebrex can promote the upregulation of cannabinoids. Studies show that cannabinoids present some benefits for cancer patients. Cannabinoids can help control chronic pain by regulating neurotransmitter activity, releasing specific neuropeptides and reducing neural inflammation.[13] They also increase appetite, which can help a cancer patient keep weight on and lower the risk of muscle mass loss. Cannabinoids are shown to improve the quality of sleep, relieve nausea as well. THC promotes apoptosis and inhibits metastasis.[14] Celebrex increases cannabinoid uptake and downregulates the production of NF-κB.

To answer the question if Oasis of Hope uses CBD or THC in our protocols, we don't. The use of cannabis products has not been legalized yet in Mexico. There is no contraindication for cannabinoid products and our protocol. We highly oppose self-medication. We urge our patients to find a medical expert trained in the use of cannabis products with cancer patients. They may use such products at home, but may not bring them to Mexico.

CANCER'S PH

Another way we can attack cancer indirectly is to take it out of its pH comfort zone. A waste product of cancer's metabolism is lactic acid. For this reason, a tumor's microenvironment is acidic. Whereas the pH environment in healthy cells is a very neutral pH environment, at about 7.4, tumors have an acidic extracellular pH around 5 to 6.6.[15] The tumor itself tends toward neutrality. Therefore, the logic would be that if we alkalinize our bodies, we could destroy or change the tumor's acidic environment. Conditions would be less conducive for cancer to thrive.

Many alkalinizing therapies were developed in the 1970s and 1980s. Few have been successful because our bodies have a buffering system that neutralizes acids or alkaline substances to maintain a stable pH no matter what. If you study the controlling mechanisms of our body, pH homeostasis is probably the most sophisticated. No matter what you eat or drink, your blood's pH is going to be stable. The body regulates pH efficiently. It is a critical function because very slight changes in our body's pH can easily result in death. The human body's normal range of pH is very narrow between 7.35 to 7.45. Dropping just below 7 is certain death without immediate medical intervention.[16] Tumors live in environments with pH levels much lower than 7 in ranges from 5-6.6. But the body must react instantly to the ingestion of acidic products to preserve its pH above 7.

Take this noteworthy example of how our pH buffering system maintains homeostasis. Coca-Cola is exceptionally acidic with a pH level of 2.37.[17] (To be fair, the pH of orange juice is 3.3 and coffee is between 5 and 6.) Though Coca-Cola is very unhealthy, drinking one bottle won't kill you. But Coke is so acidic that if you pour it in a container and attempt to bring it to a neutral pH balance of 7, you will have to dilute it with ten gallons of water. Remember, your body cannot drop below a pH of 7; so does that mean that after drinking one bottle of Coke, you will have to drink ten gallons of water or you will die? The answer is no. No one could safely consume ten gallons of water at once. Whether you drink Coke, orange juice or coffee, our body's pH does not become acidic because the buffering system neutralizes the pH immediately.

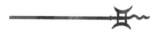

Whatever effort made to change the pH of a tumor by drinking or injecting alkaline substances will not be effective because our body neutralizes it almost immediately. We caution patients about spending four thousand dollars on an alkaline water machine if they think the water is a cancer therapy. Drinking highly alkaline water will not kill cancer.

If you look at the metabolism reserve energy bank, when you drink acidic substances, your body will buffer and neutralize them at the cost of your metabolic reserve. When you consume alkaline foods, your body is going to neutralize them, but there will be a metabolic benefit. Every time you consume alkaline foods, you are putting money into your metabolic bank. Every time you eat acidic food, you are withdrawing money from your metabolic bank. However, you cannot change your body's pH for an extended period of time. Your urine can be alkalinized, and your saliva may be acidified. But your plasma will maintain its normal pH no matter what you do. A tumor's environment is highly resistant to change.

SODIUM BICARBONATE THERAPY

Studies demonstrate that certain elements can impact the pH of the tumor's environment. Baking soda—sodium bicarbonate—seems to be the most effective. Sodium bicarbonate has not demonstrated a direct impact on cancer. Still, it may be a useful indirect attack as it has demonstrated the ability to slow the progression of cancer.[18,19] What has been somewhat controversial is how sodium bicarbonate should be administered. The discredited physician Tullio Simoncini proposed that cancer is a fungus. He claimed that tumors could be destroyed by intratumoral infusions of baking soda. Both our experience and clinical studies conclude that infusing baking soda into tumors is not effective.[20]

We haven't written off baking soda as an adjuvant cancer therapy. Recent studies suggest that oral consumption of baking soda could affect the pH of a tumor's environment. Some studies even suggest that it may help inhibit tumors metastasis.[21] Because of this evidence, we recommend that our patients drink sodium bicarbonate mixed in water daily.

**Oasis of Hope treatment protocols wage
an indirect attack on cancer.**

CONCLUSION

Conventional therapies such as chemotherapy, radiation and surgery are direct attacks on cancer. But to undermine cancer, indirect attacks can be superior. A deep understanding

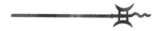

of the conditions and factors involved in the progression and proliferation of cancer has been our driving mechanism for discovering and employing medications and therapies that affect a tumor's microenvironment and metabolism. Our treatment approach wages an indirect attack on cancer.

This chapter explained the importance of downregulating the production of NF-κB. We use COX-2 inhibitors for this purpose. We discussed how hyperthermia therapy inhibits NF-κB activation,[22] cannabinoids inhibit NF-κB production, and baking soda can change the pH of a tumor's microenvironment, which could help slow cancer's growth. In the next chapter, we will show you how to punch cancer in the mouth.

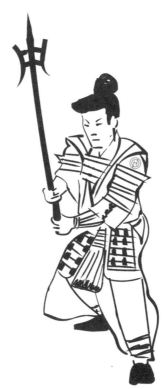

Charles Bender • Prostate Cancer • 1999

I was diagnosed with prostate cancer in 1999. I had a radical prostatectomy at Mission Hospital in California. A few months later, my cancer levels started rising, and I was told that I would need massive radiation treatments that may not even work. My father and three uncles had been to Oasis of Hope before my diagnosis and obtained excellent results. Three had prostate cancer, and one uncle had stomach cancer. When my cancer returned, with much prayer and research, my wife, Sandy, and I decided to commit to Oasis of Hope's protocol.

I have been in remission since 2000 with my PSA at the same level since then. We were blessed to have caring doctors and nurses, in a faith-based hospital, who took excellent care of me. They prayed for us during my treatment, and ever since. I have had several follow-up visits since 2000. Sandy and I call them "Tune-ups." We feel that Oasis of Hope is family. Every time we return for a follow-up visit, we feel the friendship and the love of Christ.

I would not hesitate to use Oasis of Hope's protocol again, should there be any cancer recurrence. We have also had the privilege of meeting new friends, over the years at Oasis of Hope, that have become brothers and sisters in Christ.

—Charles "Chuck" Bender
San Juan Capistrano, California
United States

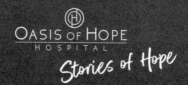

虛實

EIGHT

PUNCH WHERE IT HURTS

You may advance and be absolutely irresistible,
if you make for the enemy's weak points.

—Sun Tzu
The Art of War
Weak Points and Strong

Homer, the great mythologist, wrote *The Iliad*, a poem about the fiercest mortal warrior in history—Achilles.[1] From the day he was born, Achilles' mother Thetis was determined to make him immortal. When he was an infant, she would burn him in the fire every night and dress the wounds with magical ointment. She also submerged him in the River Styx because its waters could make a person invulnerable like the gods. The divine water touched all of his body except where Thetis held onto him, which was his heal.[2]

Achilles was unbeatable in combat. His highly skilled fighting techniques made him the Greek army's fiercest warrior. He had special impenetrable armor that protected him from every weapon. Hephaestus was the blacksmith from the heavens crafted the armor for him. Achilles was an invincible threat to every foe because no weapon could harm him. He was eventually killed, but it took the god Apollos to guide an arrow to the one place of vulnerability—Achilles' heel. The lesson we can draw from this Greek myth is that when it appears that an enemy is invincible, one must find its Achilles' heal, the place where it is weak.

Cancer has several vulnerabilities that can be used against it.

WHERE IS CANCER WEAK?

To punch cancer where it hurts, it takes more than finding its weaknesses. General Sun Tzu emphasized that one had to identify an enemy's strengths as well.[3] It is critical to gain an understanding of cancer's strengths. By learning about cancer's strengths, we can implement strategies to protect ourselves from the threats it presents. By learning about its weaknesses, we can uncover opportunities to hurt cancer.

SWOT ANALYSIS

A SWOT analysis of cancer's **S**trengths, **W**eaknesses, **O**pportunities and **T**hreats, can be quite revealing. At Oasis of Hope, we use SWOT analyses to find new ways to undermine cancer. By evaluating cancer's metabolism, we uncover how to leverage its metabolic traits against the disease's progression. Let's take a look at some of cancer's SWOT—strengths, weaknesses, opportunities and threats.

STRENGTHS

Cancerous cells have distinctive strengths compared with healthy cells. Malignant cells are highly adaptable. They can adapt quickly and powerfully to any change that takes place in the body. Malignant cells will function or reproduce despite sudden changes made in the body. Treatments like chemotherapy lose their efficacy over time because malignant cells mutate to protect themselves.

Cancerous cells release proteins via cell signaling that inactivate certain chemotherapies. Like survival of the fittest, some mutated cells have protective qualities that help them survive specific chemotherapies. Chemoresistant cells have information that resides on the surface of their cells. This epigenetic information is be passed on to new cells when they are forming. The new group of cells is resistant to the chemotherapy that had initially worked.[4] Treatment resistance warrants a dedicated chapter. We will look at it closely in chapter twelve.

Fear fuels cancer.

Another strength of cancer is fear. Fear fuels cancer. Cancer is a bully that intimidates the person who is diagnosed. It is quite common for a person to equate a cancer diagnosis with death. Some patients have expressed that they may be walking around, but feel like they are already dead.

The emotional distress that cancer provokes creates a physiological process known as the fight or flight response, in which prolonged stress diminishes the immune system's function. A depressed immune system fosters the rapid growth of malignant cells, causing a tumor to multiply at an alarming rate. In this book, we have repeatedly stated how chemotherapy and radiation devastate the immune system. But those treatments are not the only culprits. Fear, depression and anxiety are common cognitive responses to cancer-associated thoughts. Negative emotions and psychosocial distress suppress the correct function of the immune system.

We will help you overcome the cancer fear factor.

We help our patients overcome the cancer fear factor. Emotional responses to any threat are hard-wired to various organs and have pathways to elicit the fight or flight mechanism. The process is a function of the sympathoadrenal system.[5] The sympathoadrenal pathway consists of the hypothalamic-pituitary-adrenal axis, the sympathetic–adrenal–medullary axis, and the hypothalamic-pituitary-ovarian axis. When we feel fear, anxiety or depression, our adrenal glands use energy to produce and release the hormones epinephrine, norepinephrine and cortisol.[6] Epinephrine is released to constrict blood flow, which increases blood pressure and opens airways in the lungs. In this way, epinephrine helps provide enough oxygen to generate the needed energy to fight or escape the threat. The release of norepinephrine provides strength to the muscles, including the heart. Cortisol mobilizes glucose reserves to produce the burst of energy need to fight or escape.[7]

In an acute situation, the fight or flight response is critical to saving a person's life. In the case of cancer, both emotional and physical stressors could lead to a chronic state of fight or flight. This is harmful to the immune system. The body dedicates energy to producing adrenal chemicals rather than maintaining the immune system in an optimal working condition.

WEAKNESSES

Do you remember the story of the scorpion that can't swim and asks a frog to take him across a river? The frog hesitates because he doesn't want to be stung. The scorpion assures the frog he won't be stung as it would mean that both would drown. The frog agrees, and midway across the river the scorpion stings him. As they begin to sink, the frog asks why the scorpion would sting him. The scorpion replies that it is in his nature. It's ironic that it's in cancer's nature to kill its host. If cancer is not arrested, it will eventually take the life of the host it needs to survive. Cancer ultimately works against itself. This is a weakness that can be leveraged against it.

Another weakness of cancer's metabolism is that it is disorganized. Since malignant cells don't communicate with each other, they are not efficient at working together to fend off attacks. Cancer has several vulnerabilities, including being

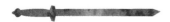

adverse to oxygen-rich environments and high heat. Another weakness is that cancer needs high amounts of glucose to produce energy and replicate.

Superfood nutrients can turn off oncogenes.

OPPORTUNITIES

By evaluating cancer's strengths and weaknesses, opportunities to undermine cancer become more apparent. There are many opportunities to modulate cancer's metabolic to punch it where it hurts! Opportunities include using food to turn oncogenes off, starving malignant cells of glucose and promoting alkalinity within the tumor's microenvironment. We utilize tumor-specific antigens from a patient's immune system as a targeted treatment. We also administer therapies that increase the level of oxygen within malignant cells. Oasis of Hope's treatment protocols have been developed to leverage all of cancer's metabolic traits against it.

THREATS

Recurrence is the number one threat cancer presents. Malignant cells are incredibly resilient and can regroup to form tumors again after a treatment cycle has destroyed most of a tumor. Almost all conventional treatments—chemotherapy, radiation and surgery—are effective initially and often take cancer into partial remission. Cancer's abilities to mutate and adapt are metabolic traits that make cancer a constant threat even after successful treatment. It also, over time, begins to limit treatment options.

Another threat cancer presents is the weakening of the immune system resulting from conventional therapies. It isn't uncommon for cancer patients to die from an unrelated illness due to their suppressed immune system. It's vital to be vigilant about all health issues when facing cancer.

PREEMPTIVE PUNCHES

We know how cancer grows, proliferates, spreads, becomes resistant and recurs. This knowledge is power. It is like a chess game. The best chess players know their opponents' historical strategic behaviors. They can predict what the opponent will do many moves in advance. Our strategic plan anticipates what cancer will do a few moves in advance based on our knowledge of cancer's metabolic traits and behavior. With this information, we can develop and administer preemptive punches. We want to hurt cancer as much as possible before it

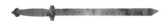

hurts our patients. Our predictive therapy design process addresses immediate, intermediate and long-term concerns. Immediate concerns include acute health issues that pose an imminent threat to our patient's life. We employ interventions to detox a patient from chemotherapy and radiation, recover the quality of life and rebuild the immune system. These efforts are necessary to obtain the time needed for the patient to receive all of the benefits of the alternative therapies we use.

Immediate concerns include digestion, respiration, pain, weight loss, anemia, potential fracturing of bones, fatigue, weakness and fluid buildup. Anything that hinders a patient from benefiting from our therapies, or represents an immediate threat to their lives, is addressed.

Intermediate concerns are centered on slowing and reversing cancer progression, inhibiting the spread, boosting the immune system, and helping the patient outlive their initial prognosis. We aim to help a person live longer with a high quality of life.

Long-term concerns are centered on recurrence and a new diagnosis with a different primary cancer. For long-term victory, lifestyle changes, especially in nutrition and stress management, are essential. Long-term strategies are all about prevention once a person has been cancer-free for five years.

NO CODE OF HONOR

Ultimately, we must never forget that cancer has no code of honor. It fights dirty and punches where it hurts the most. Whereas most illnesses progress along a predictable path, cancer will change its course in unexpected ways at unpredictable times. It's different than other conditions that way.

With most diseases, there is a clear understanding of how it will progress. Take diabetes, for example. A patient can know what their current symptoms are, what the consequences of not getting treated will be, what will happen if they get treatment, and what will certainly not happen if they get treatment. There is a fairly consistent pattern to the evolution of the disease. Most illnesses follow a textbook predictable progression, so it is straightforward to understand the course of the disease and make adjustments with anticipation.

Cancer, on the other hand, does not adhere to any textbook. It is a rule breaker. For instance, we can say that brain tumors never spread to other organs. As a rule, that is true, and for this reason, they are not staged the same way as other types of cancer.[8] As the French never say, "Il ne faut jamais dire

'Fontaine, Je ne boirai pas de ton eau,'" with cancer, never say never.

With cancer, making assumptions is not an option. We have to prepare for the unpredictable. Though we cannot predict with one hundred percent certainty, we can implement measures to reduce risks of threatening evolutions significantly. That's why, for us, the immune system is the most crucial factor.

In our experience, optimizing the immune system is far more critical than predicting cancer's behavior at all times. Your immune system is the most potent agent that protects against any foreign or abnormal cell in any part of your body. In fact, it can really deliver a preemptive punch to hit cancer where it hurts. In chapter eleven, we will go in-depth about how we effectively use immune-therapy.

Your immune system is your most potent cancer-fighting agent.

CONCLUSION

In this chapter, we talked about punching cancer where it hurts. In the next chapters, we will share the specific therapies we use to do just that. Read on to learn about our whole-body hyperthermia, amygdalin, Ozone therapy, dendritic cell vaccine and our one-two-three punch strategy to keep cancer off balance.

But before you get into the next chapter, we want to share a fundamental truth. Though we have stated that cancer is not predictable, not all surprises are bad. One of our close family members was diagnosed with lung cancer. The tumor was less than two centimeters in size, but he was considered inoperable due to other factors. He had a fragile heart, was over eighty years old and didn't want to undergo another medical procedure. Instead of invasive surgery, the doctors employed a wait and watch strategy. The tumor never grew enough to cause him any difficulties, and he lived the rest of his life without any threat from cancer. The fact that the disease did not progress in the usual way turned out to be a blessing.

Get ready to receive unexpected blessings!

STORY OF HOPE
Jenni Beer • Brainstem Glioma •2015

On September 14, 2015, my 39th birthday, I was diagnosed with a brainstem Glioma and given a year to live. I immediately began a keto no sugar diet, as well as consulting with a naturopath and starting a lot of natural supplements known to help with cancer treatment. I had radiation and chemo tablets in late 2015, with a further two rounds of the chemo tablets, but my platelets kept dropping. We were praying and researching different options.

A man from my sister's church, named Ross Kelly, was a volunteer chaplain at Oasis of Hope Hospital in Tijuana, Mexico. He called us and said he thought I should go to Oasis of Hope for treatment. This recommendation confirmed our research and felt like an answer to prayer as to which way we should go next.

I went to Oasis of Hope for the first time in May 2016. I had five further visits for treatment to Oasis of Hope. My tumor remained stable for four years and had a drastic reduction in size and no evidence of progressive disease. In November of 2019, I had a recurrence of disease, so I went back for my seventh treatment in early 2020 and am again continuing to remain stable. Oasis of Hope Hospital has been amazing for me. The treatment experience doesn't feel like the treatment you get at a regular hospital, and the friendships I've gained from my treatment visits have been so good. I still regularly keep in touch with some of the other patients I have met on my different visits. This hospital treats the whole person, and the doctors, nurses, and entire staff have been so supportive and caring along the way. I thank God that He led me to Oasis of Hope Hospital.

—Jenni Beer
Brisbane, Queensland
Australia

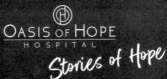

軍爭

NINE

ENGAGE WITH FORCE

The difficulty of tactical maneuvering consists in turning the devious into the direct, and misfortune into gain.

—Sun Tzu
The Art of War
Maneuvering

When my daughters were quite young, I decided that I wanted to prepare them to be safe in this world. We enrolled as a family in Taekwondo classes. We would go from their ballet classes, change uniforms and get ready for some kicking and punching. The *dojang* (school) had never seen such grace in the *poomsaes* (forms). Watching my daughters do their exercises was like watching a martial art ballet production.

If you ever trained in Taekwondo, you will know that once you have mastered some techniques and forms, you are tested to move up in belts. The final challenge of every test is to break a board with your bare hands or feet. When you watch people breaking boards, it's easy to assume that they are using special soft boards. My daughters and I found out that the boards were solid and hard to break. On a few occasions, I didn't engage the board with the right force, and the result was just what you are imagining—pain. When my four-year-old daughter had to break a board with an ax kick, I was worried that she might get hurt. She tried twice and wasn't successful. I could see a painful expression on her face and was sure she was going to cry, but her *Sabomnim* (master instructor) was sure she was going to succeed. He gave her words of encouragement and reminded her how to engage with force. He told her not to focus her power on the board, but to focus it a few inches behind the board. He also told her that the middle of the board was its weakest point, and if she would target that, she would surely break through the board. She lifted her leg high in the air, brought it down like an ax, and sliced through the board like a hot knife slicing through butter. Success!

There are precise moments in the fight against cancer when it is necessary to **engage with force**. As mentioned in previous chapters, we disagree with the conventional all-out direct attack on cancer because those tactics don't protect the patient's quality of life. Chemotherapy causes devastating collateral damage to healthy cells throughout the body. At times, its side effects cause more suffering than the disease. Cancer has natural strongholds against a direct attack. Sometimes, trying to knock it out with chemotherapy can be like hitting a brick wall.

Unlike traditional oncology, our strategy capitalizes on the cancer's weak points and applies force to where it is most vulnerable. We employ therapies that can deal a fatal blow to malignant cells, while not damaging healthy cells as chemotherapy does. This chapter will highlight two of our natural cancer killers. But first, let's talk about how we administer natural anticancer therapies to prepare a patient's body and achieve better results.

Oasis of Hope therapies deal a fatal blow to malignant cells without harming healthy cells.

PRECONDITIONING

Sun Tzu taught that it is a great challenge to convert an enemy's strengths and threats into an advantage for your army. If you can do that, you can engage the enemy with force and be much more effective. According to Sun Tzu, to turn obstacles

into an advantage requires maneuvering the army to a better position for launching the attack.

Our approach to treating cancer is revolutionary when compared to mainstream treatment methods. With chemotherapy or radiation, the patient undergoes aggressive therapy on the very first day. At Oasis of Hope, we do preconditioning to position the patient to a more favorable condition, providing a better position from where to launch the attack. We start with therapies designed to prepare the patient for the oxidative therapy we will administer on the following days. For example, we administer Ozone. Studies show that Ozone protects healthy cells from the toxicity of oxidative therapies.[1] It also combats hypoxia within tumors, making them more susceptible to treatment.

We know this is an effective tactic. A few years back, we were quite encouraged when we received a powerful affirmation of how effective our preconditioning was. We had an unexpected visit from an oncologist who runs a radiation treatment center in southern California. This doctor wanted to learn about our therapies and get to know us. On the visit, he explained how he had treated five patients, over a period of two years, that were responding exceptionally well to radiation therapy. They had done so well that he could lower the doses of radiation for these patients. The lower rads produced less intense side effects. When he investigated, he found a common denominator with all five patients—Oasis of Hope. He came to Oasis of Hope to find out what we were doing so the patients could get results with low-dose radiation. When he saw our preconditioning protocol designed to increase oxygen levels in the bloodstream and tumor, he said, "Now it makes sense. When I was specializing in oncology in the 1970s, we were told that if we could increase our patients' oxygen levels, we could lower the radiation doses. I have no idea why oncologists don't do oxygen therapies."

After our preconditioning therapies, the patient is positioned and ready to engage cancer with force. We have an oxidizing protocol that we will expand on in future chapters. Right now, let's talk about a therapy that can hit cancer right where it hurts. It works like an inside job because it uses the lack of an enzyme in malignant cells to release its cancer-killing force.

OUT WITH THE NEW & IN WITH THE OLD

We have a phenomenal research team that works hand in hand with our physicians. Combining research with clinical practice leads to some exciting breakthroughs. We make dedicated efforts to constantly evolve and discover better ways to engage cancer with force while protecting our patients' quality of life. But the saying, "out with the old, and in with the new," is not always the best thing to do. Sometimes "out with the new and in with the old" is more effective. Not everything old is obsolete. The last time we checked, air and water are still very popular with the human race. We all need to breathe and stay hydrated. Imagine a doctor telling you that air and water were obsolete! Advances in medicine can be useful, but some old, even ancient, medicines are tried and true. We don't throw something out just because it is old.

We started using our very first alternative cancer treatment back in 1963, and guess what? We still use it today. Studies conducted as recently as 2019 confirm its multiple anticancer therapeutic actions. Yes, we are talking about amygdalin, also known as laetrile and Vitamin B17. We are proud that our founder, Dr. Ernesto Contreras, Sr., was the first doctor in Mexico to use amygdalin. All of the clinics in Mexico that use it have Dr. Contreras, Sr. to thank. Amygdalin's use goes back further than 1963. It was first used as a cancer treatment in 1845 in Russia, and the USA in the 1920s.[2] It came to prominence in the 1950s when it was first called "laetrile." The medical establishment completely dismissed it in the 1960s and

1970s. It is as controversial now as it was then. Amygdalin's opponents point to the lack of clinical studies. Proponents allege that studies in the past were rigged and done to prove amygdalin useless.

When considering the validity of amygdalin, follow the science. Data is better than controversy. The resurgence in the scientific community's interest in amygdalin has generated many studies that have been published in top peer-reviewed medical journals. *Cancer Medicine* published a study in May 2019 that stated, "Amygdalin is known to have an anti-tumor effect in solid tumors such as lung cancer, bladder cancer and renal cell carcinoma by affecting cell cycle, inducing apoptosis and cytotoxicity, and regulating immune function."[3]

We are pleased that the US National Library of Medicine has made this study available online at https://www.ncbi.nlm.nih.gov/pmc/articles/PMC6558459/. We are displeased with Google's policies that ban advertising from organizations that publish information about amygdalin. (Can somebody say Big Pharma? Or Big Brother?) There could be a whole book on the efforts to suppress information on amygdalin and other alternative therapies. This book, however, is sharing the scientific evidence of alternative cancer treatments and the Oasis of Hope strategies designed for undermining cancer.

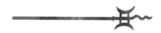

LET'S CLEAR UP THE NAME CONFUSION

At Oasis of Hope, we use amygdalin, the natural medicine derived from apricot pits. "Laetrile" was the name given by Dr. Ernest Krebs, Jr., in 1949, for the product created when he put amygdalin through a synthetic process to purify it. The name "laetrile" combines the words "laevorotatory" and "mandelonitrile," referring to its molecular structure.

Krebs' intrigue with amygdalin was based on his interest in the Hunza people's longevity who live in the Himalayas in the northernmost part of Pakistan. The Hunza are known for longevity. Some of their people live up to one hundred and thirty-five years.

Krebs noted that the incidence of cancer in the Hunza was extremely low. He observed that the mainstays in their diet included apricots, the bitter almond from the apricot pit, raw nuts, lima beans, sorghum and clover. All of these foods are sources of amygdalin. Krebs theorized that the amygdalin in the bitter almond was a vitamin missing in most people's diets. Amygdalin's structure is similar to a B vitamin. That's why Krebs called it *Vitamin B17*. It is not recognized as a vitamin by the American Institute of Nutrition Vitamins.[4] We agree that amygdalin is not technically a vitamin. By definition, a vitamin is something the body requires to maintain health, and in its absence, death will eventually result. Humans can survive without amygdalin. Whether you call Amygdalin laetrile or vitamin B17, its anticancer qualities are what is important.

AN INSIDE JOB

Amygdalin can engage cancer with force. It's quite fascinating that amygdalin's fight against tumors works like an inside job because it uses one of cancer's traits to attack tumors. Amygdalin releases cyanide within malignant cells when metabolized. Amygdalin's cyanide radical is its primary cancer-killing mechanism.[5] Cyanide is only released within the tumor. That's why we say it is an inside job. Healthy cells have a protective enzyme called rhodanese. Rhodanese prevents the release of cyanide within normal cells. Cancerous cells do not have rhodanese. Amygdalin is innocuous to healthy cells but can be lethal to malignant cells. In sharp contrast to chemotherapy that kills cancer and healthy cells alike, amygdalin only kills malignant cells and provides additional benefits to patients.[6]

USE OF AMYGDALIN IS EVIDENCE-BASED

Critics of amygdalin point to the lack of evidence of its efficacy as a cancer treatment. They often argue that all case

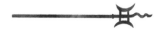

studies are anecdotal and have not been conducted in a scientific method. The best way to diffuse this criticism is to provide evidence published in peer-reviewed medical journals. We are pleased that there are many published studies, and more are in process. Let us take a look at the cancer-fighting qualities of amygdalin the studies have found.

AMYGDALIN INHIBITS ANGIOGENESIS

A plan to control cancer starts with understanding how tumors grow. Angiogenesis is the formation of new blood vessels. Cancer cells, like healthy cells, require blood to supply them with glucose to keep growing. As a tumor grows larger, its center tends to get cut off from its blood supply. The tumor sends out angiogenic factors that provoke the formation of new blood vessels. Without angiogenesis, it is tough for cancer to progress. If a tumor can stimulate the formation of hundreds of new capillaries, it can grow without limitations.[7] Inhibiting angiogenesis is key to controlling the growth of cancer, or even killing it. A study found that amygdalin has angiogenesis inhibitory effects.[8] This anti-tumor effect should be evidence enough to include amygdalin in the treatment of cancer. But amygdalin possesses many more anticancer qualities. Read on.

AMYGDALIN INDUCES APOPTOSIS

Apoptosis—programmed cell death—is the mechanism by which every cell's life ends at the right time. Space is then made for a replacement cell. Tumors have genes that suppress apoptosis. The absence of apoptosis is why cancer cells are virtually immortal and that much more challenging to kill. Fortunately, several nutrients can induce apoptosis in cancer cells. In 2012, a study in China identified how amygdalin induces apoptosis.[9] The study was conducted on human cell lines of cervical cancer. It was observed that amygdalin downregulates the anti-apoptotic protein Bcl-2 and upregulates the pro-apoptotic Bax protein. Before this study, amygdalin was thought to work via necrosis alone, when in fact, it also works through apoptosis.

AMYGDALIN HINDERS METASTASES

Dr. Sugiura is not the only researcher who uncovered amygdalin's ability to hinder metastases. In 2014, researchers in Germany conducted an in vitro study on the effects of amygdalin on bladder cancer cells. They observed that "Amygdalin alters the migratory behavior of tumor cells."[10] This finding supports the use of amygdalin because most cancer

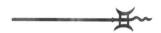

deaths result from metastases, not the primary tumor. For long-term survival, it is critical to prevent or control metastases.

AMYGDALIN EXERTS ANTI-INFLAMMATORY & ANALGESIC EFFECTS

A study was conducted in 2013 by researchers at the Second University of Naples, Italy and the Department of Chemical Engineering at the University in Barcelona, Spain. The study found that amygdalin suppresses the gene expression that promotes the inflammatory response.[11] Another study conducted in Korea in 2007 concluded that "Amygdalin exerts anti-inflammatory and analgesic effects."[12] These findings are significant as the inflammation response may provide an increase in the availability of new blood vessels that can feed tumor growth.

A favorable side effect of amygdalin is pain control. Its analgesic effect allows us to transition patients away from addictive painkillers or reduce the dose. Amygdalin is so effective at pain control that it is registered as an analgesic in Mexico. Amygdalin has earned its place at Oasis of Hope just for its pain control quality. Its numerous anticancer qualities are priceless added values.

INHIBITOR OF LUNG CANCER CELL PROLIFERATION

In 2004, researchers in China conducted a study that demonstrated that amygdalin inhibits the proliferation of lung cancer cells.[13] This is noteworthy as thirty-one years previously, Memorial Sloan Kettering's Dr. Sugiura concluded that amygdalin inhibited lung metastases. The scientific method consists of observation and the ability to repeat results when using the same procedure. Ongoing studies demonstrate amygdalin's effect on stabilizing tumors and slowing growth, just like the study published in *Cancer Medicine* in May of 2019. Considering the body of evidence of amygdalin's anticancer actions these studies present, we call on the FDA and the NCI to embrace it.

Oasis of Hope has administered amygdalin to tens of thousands of cancer patients since 1963. We have determined amygdalin to be completely safe and effective. We are hopeful that cancer research on the use of amygdalin will continue and that in the future, the body of evidence will obligate the FDA to approve it for cancer treatment in the USA.

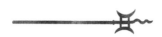

THE NEED FOR ALTERNATIVES TO CHEMOTHERAPY

On December 23, 1971, President Richard Nixon signed "The National Cancer Act," Senate Bill 1828 (SB1829).[1] This legislation was America's declaration of war on cancer. SB1828 allowed cancer research funding to be approved directly by the President of the United States, bypassing normal channels and processes for budget approval. Unfortunately, the increase in funding was surpassed by the rise in cancer incidence and mortality. In 1970, the number of annual cancer deaths reached 407,000 Americans.[15] Fast forward to 2020, forty-nine years after the war on cancer was declared, annual cancer deaths in America will surpass 607,000.[16]

There is some good news to report. According to the American Cancer Society, cancer deaths in both men and women have declined by twenty-six percent since it peaked in 1991.[17] But this reduction is attributed to the decrease of tobacco use and early detection, not the improvement in cancer treatment. Though the mortality rate has declined, the absolute number of cancer deaths continues to grow each year, as does the population.

Another number that continues to go up is spending on new drug development. The Tufts Center for the Study of Drug Development has documented that the cost to develop, test and register a single new cancer drug has risen to more than $2.7 billion.[18] The high cost of drug development explains in part why new drugs such as Opdivo, Keytruda, Kadcyla and Afinitor, which can cost $10,000.00-$100,000.00 per treatment. Kymriah, a leukemia drug, costs upwards of $475,000.00 for one month of treatment.[19]

While new cancer drugs promise better results, at least in the first four to six months of treatment, many patients cannot pay for them. Insurance companies and Medicare frequently deny payment of such expensive medication.

It is a misconception that Medicare covers all medication. Medicare limits coverage. Its policy states, "Your doctor or other healthcare provider may recommend you get services more often than Medicare covers. Or, they may recommend services that Medicare does not cover. If this happens, you may have to pay some or all of the costs. It's important to ask questions so you understand why your doctor is recommending certain services and whether Medicare will pay for them."[20] The exorbitant cost of new targeted therapies continues to make treatment inaccessible to large segments of the population.

The United Kingdom's National Health System (NHS) has published a list of twenty-five chemotherapies it will not cover.

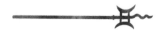

The NHS states that to provide expensive new cancer drugs, it would have to cut other healthcare from its budget.[21] Access to such drugs is on a private pay basis. Only the wealthy can access the newer, more expensive chemotherapies. If new drugs are financially inaccessible, are there affordable treatment options that compare to expensive wonder drugs?

We use a natural alternative to expensive chemotherapies—ascorbate (Vitamin C). High-Dose Intravenous Vitamin C (HDIVC) is affordable and has proved to be safe and effective. Let us take a close look at the scientific evidence supporting the use of HDIVC to treat cancer patients.

FIRST USE OF HDIVC

The National Cancer Institute reports that in 1972, Dr. Ewan Cameron and Dr. Andrew Campbell were the first doctors to study the use of Vitamin C for treating cancer. In 1976, they teamed up with Nobel Prize Laureate Dr. Linus Pauling to conduct clinical trials. It was found that the blood serum level Vitamin C needed to produce anticancer effects could not be achieved via oral administration. The study found that administration of high dose intravenous Vitamin C (HDIVC) could reach the blood serum levels necessary to produce death in cancer cells. The NCI states, "Research suggests that pharmacologic concentrations of ascorbate, such as those achieved with IV administration, may result in cell death in many cancer cell lines."[22]

THE OPPOSITION

Every promising cancer treatment meets with opposition by those who do not believe in its value. Some researchers will invest time in discrediting a therapy. HDIVC is no exception. The first argument against the use of intravenous Vitamin C is that most of the studies have been conducted in vitro, and there is a lack of in vivo studies. In February 2015, a group of researchers published their systematic review of studies on HDIVC in the prestigious journal *The Oncologist*.[23] They reiterated the well-established fact that oral Vitamin C has no anti-tumor effect. The group went on to say that there was a lack of double-blind studies (in vivo) to provide sufficient evidence that intravenous Vitamin C possesses anti-tumor qualities, lowers chemo-toxicity or enhances chemotherapy. To sum up their argument, researchers accept that HDIVC kills cancer cells in vitro, but they want to see more studies done in humans.

The second objection to the use of HDIVC is that the mechanism of action is not well defined. A study published in

Frontiers in Oncology in 2014 reported that "The majority of investigations to date concluded that increased ascorbate [Vitamin C] led to decreased tumor growth, but data on mechanisms and dose are inconclusive."[24] To sum up this argument, scientists state that HDIVC is effective, but it should not be used because the precise mechanism of how it kills cancer is unknown.

Let us point out that in both arguments against HDIVC, the studies acknowledge that intravenous Vitamin C does kill cancer cells. The studies are focused on details that do not discredit HDIVC as a viable anticancer agent.

To address these two arguments, let us review several patient cases that have been published by the NCI and others. We will also share with you the results of several studies on the mechanism of action of HDIVC.

CLINICAL CASES OF HDIVC USE IN HUMANS

Several researchers, including Mark Levine of the National Cancer Institute (NCI), have reviewed a number of patient cases utilizing the *NCI Best Case Series Guidelines*. After completing their review, they concluded, "In light of recent clinical pharmacokinetic findings and in vitro evidence of anti-tumor mechanisms, these case reports indicate that the role of high-dose intravenous Vitamin C therapy in cancer treatment should be reassessed."[25] In other words, the researchers acknowledge that HDIVC should not be dismissed, but rather should be considered more carefully. Let us look at three case studies published in the aforementioned white paper by Levine and his collaborators.

CASE STUDIES

Patient 1: Renal cell carcinoma with lung metastases

A woman diagnosed with a tumor in her kidney that had spread to the lungs was treated with HDIVC. CT scans verified that there was tumor regression in the pulmonary metastasis and the kidney.

Patient 2: Cancer of the bladder

A male patient with a primary tumor of the bladder with satellite tumors around it had part of his bladder removed. HDIVC therapy and supplements were administered. Nine years after diagnosis, the patient was found to be in good health with no recurrence or metastasis.

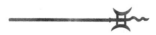

Patient 3: Lymphoma

A female patient was diagnosed with lymphoma in January 1995. The patient underwent a five-week course of radiation followed by two treatments of HDIVC per week for two months. She then took HDIVC treatment every two to three months until December 1996, at which time there was no sign of lymphoma or metastasis. In 2006, the patient continued in good health with no recurrence. She never received chemotherapy or additional radiation therapy.

Breast Cancer

Another patient case was published in the *Journal of Orthomolecular Medicine* in 2017. A patient was with metastatic breast cancer received HDIVC. After three months of treatment, the patient's tumor markers improved. The metastases to her bones and lungs were no longer present according to a PET scan. The patient opted for HDIVC because previous chemotherapy was no longer an option. She went into full remission after treatment with HDIVC.[26]

Hepatic Cancer with Lung Metastasis

A patient with primary cancer of the liver with metastasis to the lungs also responded to HDIVC. In this case, published in the *Yonsei Medical Journal,* the female patient refused chemotherapy after it had failed to reduce the metastasis in the lungs. After taking HDIVC twice a week over an extended period, the lung metastasis showed a complete regression.[27]

SAFE AND EFFECTIVE

In these four cases, it is clear that HDIVC is both safe and effective. Researchers at Wichita State University in Kansas (WSU) published a review of patient cases collected over sixteen years who had received HDIVC. They also concluded that intravenous Vitamin C administered in high doses is both safe and effective. The researchers reported that their data represented "194,054 grams, or 427 pounds, of IV Vitamin C administered to two hundred and seventy-five patients with no sign of serious kidney disease, or any other significant side effects."[28] The findings at WSU are consistent with the experience we have had at Oasis of Hope Hospital in treating thousands of patients over the last six decades.

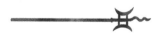

THE THERAPEUTIC MECHANISM OF HDIVC

It may be surprising, but HDIVC's primary cancer-killing mechanism is the same as some chemotherapy agents and all types of radiation—oxidative stress. Dr. Ananya Mandal defines oxidative stress as "Essentially an imbalance between the production of free radicals and the ability of the body to counteract or detoxify their harmful effects through neutralization by antioxidants."[29] HDIVC produces a cancer-killing effect via a pro-oxidative mechanism.[30] Many cancer cells have a very low content of the antioxidant enzyme catalase. As a result, malignant cells struggle to defend against oxidative stress induced by HDIVC.[31] HDIVC has a selective killing effect.[32] In some cases, HDIVC kills cancer as effectively as chemotherapy and radiation without harming healthy cells like conventional cancer treatments do.

Researchers have identified a mechanism by which HDIVC promotes a cancer-killing effect. HDIVC is a prodrug for the delivery of hydrogen peroxide (H_2O_2) to tumors, which induces cytotoxicity and cell death.[33] Tumor oxygenation unleashes HDIVC's full potential of producing hydrogen peroxide. We do this at Oasis of Hope by administering Ozone as a part of our pre-conditioning protocol mentioned earlier in this chapter.

HDIVC AND OZONE: A REAL CANCER KILLER COMBO

Solid tumors are both hypoxic and acidic.[34] Tumors that are low in ascorbate (Vitamin C) levels have an increased level of hypoxia-inducible factor (HIF).[35] HIF upregulates gene expressions that provide cancer cells with metabolic and survival advantages within most tumors' low oxygen environments. By increasing the level of Vitamin C in tumors, HIF can be downregulated. This downregulation opens the doorway to tumor oxygenation. For Vitamin C to promote oxidative stress, it must be supplied with oxygen. When Ozone is introduced into the bloodstream of a patient, it causes a cascade effect. Studies have demonstrated that Ozone autohemotherapy (O_3-AHT) lowers tumor hypoxia and helps to inhibit a tumor's aggressive behavior.[36] O_3-AHT increases the overall level of oxygenation. Increased availability of oxygen facilitates Vitamin C's production of hydrogen peroxide (H_2O_2). When H_2O_2 is formed in the fluids surrounding a tumor, it diffuses into the cancer cells and kills them by damaging their ability to synthesize DNA.

In recent years, Mark Levine of the National Cancer Institute and researchers at the Integrative Medicine Center at the University of Kansas have led the way to further investigation and study of the efficacy of HDIVC for treating

cancer patients. Their findings are consistent with our fifty-seven plus years of experience administering HDIVC to thousands of patients. Studies conducted in Belgium, Brazil, Chile, Canada, Germany, Italy, Korea and New Zealand confirm that High-Dose Intravenous Vitamin C in the treatment of cancer:

- Is safe[37]
- Is effective. In multiple clinical trials, HDIVC increases progression-free and overall survival. [38]
- Produces an anti-inflammatory effect by inhibiting pro-inflammatory cytokines[39]
- May eradicate cancer stem cells[40]
- Improves appetite, fatigue, depression and sleep cycles in patients taking chemotherapy concurrently[41]
- Selectively kills cancer cells[32]
- Has demonstrated objective results (tumor reduction) in patients who discontinued chemotherapy and opted for HDIVC[26]

Considering the evidence of the efficacy of HDIVC along with our decades of successful use, Oasis of Hope will continue to utilize this safe and effective alternative to chemotherapy for the long term.

CONCLUSION

In previous chapters, we have focused on specific therapies that leverage cancer's metabolic traits against it without making a direct attack. In this chapter, we have shared the scientific evidence of two therapies—amygdalin and HDIVC—

that directly attack tumors. We are quite confident in the safety and efficacy of these two treatments. They are excellent and are viable alternatives to chemotherapy. They work as if they were natural chemotherapies. The great advantage these cancer killers offer is that they engage the enemy with force while not provoking collateral damage to healthy cells.

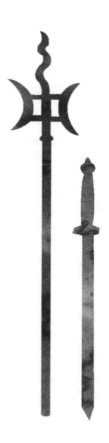

STORY OF HOPE

Michelle Tucker • Breast Cancer, Metastasis in Pancreas • 1990

I am a three-time breast cancer and pancreatic cancer warrior. I have been blessed to be a mom to three amazing children, RN for my career path, and I have mastered the art of being a tattoo artist who believes in giving back to my fellow sisters and brothers who have endured mastectomy surgery by tattooing back the areola.

I am a three-time survivor of breast cancer IDC, otherwise known as "Invasive Ductal Carcinoma" Stage 3, BRCA+. My first scare was back when I was 19. Yes, just 19 years young. My nipple inverted and began to drain a black substance from the center. I underwent a lumpectomy and took only a few weeks of oral chemo at that time. I continued with my life, career and had children. You know how it goes. You are in the midst of life and then boom, you have a funny feeling in your gut, and you follow that and make a doctor's appointment. I believe we have to be an advocate for ourselves.

Fast forward to my mid 30's. I had just moved to Arizona. It was a busy time in my life. I was doing a balancing act when I received a call early in the am that I had breast cancer stage 3. I underwent a partial mastectomy and began my treatment that consisted of radiation treatments five days a week, followed by two years of intense IV chemotherapy treatments. I lost my hair, sense of taste, and gained a high sense of smell. I was blessed to beat that battle and was put on Tamoxifen. I was told to stay on this for five years. I made it to 3.5 years on this medication until I had a PET SCAN follow up test. Then, in my late 30's, I found myself back in the chemotherapy arena once again. I opted for a full bilateral mastectomy under my surgeon and oncologist's recommendation because my cancer was in my other breast. A few months later, I had a hysterectomy, again with the stern recommendation of my oncologist. It's by the grace of GOD and His will that I beat that. I was in remission for almost three years at that time.

Fast-forwarding to December of 2016, once again, cancer returned. This time it was pancreatic CA that metastasized from my previous cancer. I followed my cancer chemotherapy regimen from my doctor. I received IV chemotherapy every twenty-one or so days, depending on my blood work. In July of 2018, my oncologist called me into his office, after my chemo treatment, and told me there was nothing else they could do for me. My tests and blood work showed evidence that I was not doing well. He looked me in the eye and said, "Michelle, I am giving you 30 days at best. Go home, get your affairs in order and live your last days." He ordered a hospice evaluation and sent me on my way. As I walked out of his office, I turned to him and said, "SEE YOU IN 30." I went home devastated, to say the least, not knowing how to tell my children. I decided to take a hot bath and pray to God for some insight. I prayed to GOD for a message.

During my bath, I heard a voice in my head telling me to look for alternative treatment options in Mexico. I followed that message and jumped out of the bath immediately and Googled alternate cancer treatments. I remember it taking longer than usual for the info to populate on my computer. When it loaded, my computer landed on OASIS OF HOPE. I filled out the form with a paragraph summary of my journey to date, and 15 minutes later, my phone rang, and I was asked to send more info.

I flew to Mexico a few days later. As I walked through the doors, I felt an overwhelming peace that takes over your spirit immediately! It's as if a flood washes over you. At that very moment, I knew I was no longer alone in this though I had walked through the doors of Oasis of Hope alone. It's so hard to put into words how Oasis of Hope makes you feel the moment you walk in the door. The ENTIRE staff makes you feel as if you are their family! The patients come from around the world to seek treatment at Oasis of Hope, and they become your family.

The treatment at Oasis of Hope is barred none the best in the world. Dr. Contreras and colleagues speak to you as a person, not a cancer patient. There is no white coat syndrome here. I mean, who else runs up to their oncology team and HUGS them? The treatment room itself has large glass windows and is beautiful, letting in plenty of natural light. It is welcoming, and turns the memory of scary treatment rooms from other clinics into peaceful serenity. They teach you how to eat correctly, cook, shop for food, decipher ingredients, and live a healthy long life with cancer.

In the treatment room, they remind you to lean on GOD, open your heart, and praise Him even in the darkness. I'm proof of that. It's been TWO years in August, 2020, since I was given 30 days to live. I went to Oasis of Hope in August 2020 for evaluation and the studies showed that I am in complete remission. Just like a marathon, you have to keep your mind focused and be strong. Cancer isn't a sprint.....it's a marathon.

—Michelle Tucker, Cancer Warrior
Queen Creek, Arizona
United States

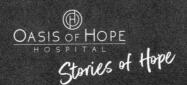

九變

TEN

CHANGE IT UP

The general who thoroughly understands the advantages
that accompany variation of tactics knows
how to handle his troops.

—Sun Tzu
The Art of War
Variation In Tactics

Nolan Ryan is one of the greatest pitchers that ever played baseball. His twenty-seven-year career is chalked full of records starting with being the player who had the longest career. No other pitcher in history has matched his strike-out record of 5,714[1] batters and seven no-hitters.[2] He threw the fastest pitch ever, blistering through the air at 108 miles per hour![3] But it wasn't his fastball that won the historic game on June 1, 1973.

Ryan was pitching for the Anaheim Angels and needed one final out for the win and to set a career-high of four no-hitters.

He was up against the Orioles second baseman Bobby Grich, who was no slouch with his career 224 home runs.[4] Grich was a great fastball hitter. Everyone was on the edge of their seats. It was a full count, three balls two strikes. It came down to one pitch. Could Grich handle Ryan's heat? Would Grich homer Ryan's fireball fastball, or would he get smoked? What came next was unexpected and beyond Grich's ability to calculate.

The capacity crown witnessed a powerful swing and a miss. Nolan Ryan struck Bobby Grich out for his 100th win. It was also Ryans fourth no-hitter, matching Sandy Koufax's record. How did Ryan outsmart Grich? He varied his tactics. He didn't send his near unhittable fastball. He threw a changeup, an off-speed pitch that comes across the plate at a much slower speed. He was a changeup master.[5] Going up against Ryan was difficult because he would toggle between his fastball, changeup and an incredible slider. Ryan knew that to win, he couldn't keep doing the same thing over and over again. To win, he needed to keep his opponent guessing.

In this chapter, we will cover a few different subjects that all tie to the theme of changing up treatments to keep cancer off balance. We will start off by explaining the positive changes that have been made in surgery, radiation and chemotherapy, and changes that still need to be made. We will end the chapter sharing about the most effective treatment strategies we use to change it up on cancer, and keep it guessing and vulnerable to our attacks.

INSANITY IN ONCOLOGY

Albert Einstein may have been the genius who declared, "Insanity is doing the same thing over and over again and expecting a different result."[6] Oxford dictionary defines insanity as extreme foolishness or irrationality.[7] At Oasis of Hope, we define insanity as insisting on using aggressive chemotherapy, radiation or surgery when the treatment is no longer helping a patient, and it's destroying their immune system and quality of life. When a treatment is no longer working, the sane thing to do is to change it up. Patients would benefit greatly if clinical oncologists and pharmaceutical companies applied that logic to conventional treatments. The time to make changes in cancer treatment is now.

POSITIVE CHANGES NEEDED

President Franklin D. Roosevelt signed the National Cancer Act on August 5, 1937, to establish the National Cancer Institute as the primary cancer research organization in the United

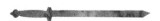

States.[8] For the next thirty years, cancer rates increased at alarming rates. In response to the cry of the American public, President Richard Nixon signed the National Cancer Act on December 23, 1971, to significantly increase cancer research funding. The war on cancer was declared and it was predicted that the cure would be found in under ten years. In 2021, it will be the 50th anniversary of the war on cancer. What has been the result of concerted cancer research and treatment efforts over the last five decades? It's easy to get lost in the interpretation of the statistics done by special interest groups, but let's look at the hard published data. In 1971, at the start of the war on cancer, an estimated 665,000 Americans were diagnosed with cancer, and 350,000 died of cancer that year in the United States.[9] Approximately three million people were alive and dealing with cancer in 1973.[10] Fast forward to the year 2020, nearly five decades later. The National Cancer Institute estimates that 1,762,450 Americans will be diagnosed with cancer this year, 606,880 will die, and there are a total of 15,338,988 people currently living with cancer in the USA.[11]

Changes must be made in cancer interventions, treatment approach, drugs and technology.

One fact research organizations point out when fundraising is that cancer is more survivable now than ever. Survivability has increased for one reason—improvements in early detection. The tragic fact that cancer deaths are up from 350,000 in 1971 to 606,880 in 2020, points to one simple truth—positive changes need to be made in conventional oncology treatment methods, drugs and technology. To continue treating cancer the same way oncologists have for the last ninety years and expect different results, is truly the definition of insanity. It is high time to change it up.

Some cancer treatment has evolved for the better over the last three to four decades. The reason driving positive change in cancer treatment is the sad reality that therapies haver become so aggressive that patients cannot tolerate them.

Patients are no longer following oncologists blindly. They are demanding a change and looking for alternatives to toxic and ineffective therapies. A treatment, even if it is the best cancer killer ever, is not viable if it destroys a patient's quality of life, or results in the patient's death. In the case of many conventional oncology treatments, patients cannot physically tolerate the toxicity, or they are aware that the benefits are far outweighed by the loss of quality of life and opt for alternatives. Before we disregard traditional cancer trearments, let's take a

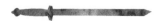

look at some positive changes being made in radiotherapy, surgery and chemotherapy.

RADIOTHERAPY

Radiotherapy was the most aggressive in the 1950s and 1960s when whole-body radiation used technology such as Cobalt teletherapy. Positive changes began in the 1970s as previous practices were discontinued. The risk of excessive radiation to surrounding tissue and the difficulty of containing the radiation source motivated changes.[12]

When healthy tissue is burned in the process of getting rid of a tumor, the damage from such burns may be irreversible. Take radiation of the cervix. Radiotherapy is exceptionally effective in cervical cancer, but it usually results in burning the rectum, small intestine or bladder. Due to that, patients will suffer proctitis, inflammation of the rectum and anus, for life. Fortunately, new radiotherapy technology has reduced the burning of surrounding tissues significantly.

NEGATIVE SIDE EFFECTS OF RADIATION

Because of the burn and production of many chemicals released by the dying cells caused by radiotherapy, there will be side effects like nausea and vomiting. The toxicity from necrotic tissue causes these symptoms. So even if a patient is not having chemotherapy, toxicity of cells killed by radiotherapy frequently induces nausea and vomiting. Necrotic tissue is dead or devitalized tissue. Adverse side effects can be more intense from necrotic tissue toxicity than from radiation and chemotherapy treatments.

Whole-body radiation, as it used to be administered, would occasionally result in a patient's death because their lungs or small intestines would be burned beyond repair. The side effects and collateral damage to healthy tissue from electron accelerators was unacceptable. Manufacturers committed to developing better technology. The first proton accelerators were proposed in the mid-1940s. They came into use in the 1970s. They were able to target tumors with great precision. According to clinical studies, "Proton beam therapy may improve the survival rate of patients by improving the local tumor treatment rate, while reducing injury to normal organs, resulting in fewer radiation-induced adverse effects. Compared with conventional photon radiotherapy, the heavier subatomic particles can deliver their energy more precisely to the tumor, with less scattering to surrounding tissues."[13]

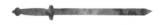

Intensity Modulated Radiation Therapy (IMRT) is another high precision computer-controlled linear accelerator. Three Dimensional Conformal Radiation Therapy (3d-CRT) uses CT, or MRI, to define the shape, size and location of tumors to deliver radiation to targeted cells, and avoid surrounding organs. These new technologies have been effective in reducing the collateral damage caused by radiation therapies. The positive change in radiotherapy has been the development of precision in targeting cancer cells only, and reducing damage to surrounding healthy tissue. But, there is another significant factor that could revolutionize the practice radiotherapy.

Oasis of Hope has changed up radiotherapy on cancer. First of all, we only recommend radiotherapy in very few cases. For example, we recommend it to patients who have bone metastases. Radiotherapy is the best way to harden fragile areas of the bone to prevent fracture. It is also very effective at controlling pain in the bones.

Here is a fascinating story that illustrates how our therapeutic changeups make a difference in the radiation cancer treatment arena. About nine years ago, we received a call from a clinical oncologist from Irvine, California. Whenever our patients needed radiotherapy, we would refer the patient to him because he was the best in town. He called to set up a visit to Oasis of Hope because he had heard a lot about it from the patients we had referred to him. We happily accepted his visit the next week. When he saw how we were using oxygen therapy, he was impressed, and explained the motive for his visit. He shared that five of his patients, was able administer lower doses of radiation and still get good results. He looked at the patients' files and discovered that they were all Oasis of Hope patients.

He clarified he could reduce dosing only for our patients. He was intrigued and wanted to find out why this was the case.He was not surprised to find out that we did oxygen therapy. According to him, back in the 1960s, when he was doing his specialty in clinical oncology, it was standard to use oxygen therapy before radiation. The method they used was hyperbaric oxygen, but it was costly back then because the hyperbaric chambers were the size of a room. Oxygenating patients before radiotherapy was discarded due to a lack of access to hyperbaric chambers. But even when the machines got smaller and relatively inexpensive, conventional therapy failed to pick up that practice again. They also failed to implement Ozone therapy, which can be even cheaper and more effective than hyperbaric oxygen. The doctor said he had always known that oxygenating patients would help lower radiation dosages. Wow!

It was a conventional radiation oncologist that made the statement, not an alternative medicine doctor.

Ozone autohemotherapy is the standard of care at Oasis of Hope.

It begs the question of why oxygen preconditioning is not the standard of care before radiotherapy? At Oasis of Hope, Ozone therapy is the standard of care. Many things are known to be effective cancer treatment practices, but they are not done for financial reasons or peer pressure. Many oncologists criticize alternative medicine as non-scientific. Fortunately, the data is not on the side of old school oncologists. We arrest the false belief that alternatives are not scientific with clinical studies published in peer-reviewed medical journals. Every single treatment we administer at Oasis of Hope is research based. The references of the clinical studies that support our treatment modalities are listed at back of the book. We encourage you to review them. Be warned that if you get into them, it will take you months to read all of the studies. There is a vast amount of scientific data supporting Oasis of Hope's cancer treatments.

SURGERY

Thank God surgical techniques and criteria are changing significantly. If you were aware of how aggressive surgeries were in the past, you would be shocked. Forty years ago, many cancer surgeries were massive and aggressive. We are dumfounded that several inhumane procedures are still performed. Thankfully they are rarely done. The most radical surgery is the trans-lumbar amputation, more commonly known as a hemicorporectomy. What is that, you ask? Let's break down the word from the Greek root words:

Hemi: Half. From Greek hemi—half.
Corpo: Body. From Latin corpus—body.
Ectomy: Surgical removal. From Greek ektomia—a cutting out of.
Put all together—hemicorporectomy: Half body surgical removal.

A hemicorporectomy (HC) is an amputation of the bottom half of a person's body. The HC was first proposed in 1950 as a curative measure for cancer in the pelvis. The first one was attempted in 1960. The patient survived for eleven days after the horrible surgery and then died.[14] Further procedures were done until the technique was improved, and patients would survive for years. In 2009, sixty-six HCs had been performed, which resulted in fifty-three percent of the patients having long-term survival.[15] Unfortunately, undergoing an HC is emotionally devastating as patients grieve the loss of half of

their bodies. Feelings of social isolation, vulnerability, poor body image and a significant decrease in self-esteem are common.[16] Considering that the prognosis of an HC is a fifty-three percent probability of long-term survival with a one hundred percent probability of emotional trauma, we call for surgeons to cease performing this uncompassionate procedure.

In breast surgery, it was common to remove both breasts, chest muscles, and part of the rib cage. Such practices harm the quality of life. In neck surgery, sometimes, the voice box is removed. Not being able to speak again harms the quality of life. In colon cancer, sometimes the rectum has to be removed, and the patient will end up with a colostomy for life. A colostomy connects the colon to the abdomen wall through an ostomy. This opening is where the stool is continuously excreted into a bag. When full, the bag must be discharged. Quality of life is obviously diminished, but some patients learn how to control their discharge and don't have to wear the bag at all times. Sometimes, death is imminent if aggressive surgery is not performed.

Patients' refusals to undergo radical surgical practices have been a catalyst for developing better techniques and surgical tools to perform less invasive procedures. At Oasis of Hope, we avoid aggressive cancer surgeries for two reasons: 1) We champion the quality of life of our patients, 2) Clinical studies show that less invasive surgeries are often as effective, or more effective than aggressive surgeries. Our changeup on surgery is that we take a conservative approach instead of an aggressive stance.

For example, clinical studies indicate that a lumpectomy in early-stage breast cancer has a cure rate equal to that of a mastectomy. A lumpectomy preserves the quality of life because the patient doesn't experience the loss of an entire breast. A study in 2019 confirmed this, and explained that the reason why a mastectomy is not more effective is that breast cancer is a systemic problem, not localized.[17]

The Oasis of Hope surgery changeup plays out in the way that we perform organ-preserving minimally invasive surgeries to protect the quality of life. In advanced-stage cancer, sometimes, a mastectomy is necessary. Even in those cases, we take care not to remove more of the body than necessary. We also do our best to perform breast reconstruction as a means to promote quality of life.

AGGRESSIVE VS. CONSERVATIVE SURGERY

A few years ago, we had a patient who was a young woman with a tumor on the back of her leg, the size of a football. She had consulted with several surgical oncologists, and they all recommended amputation of the leg up through the pelvis. The patient came to us, and we did a complete medical evaluation that took into consideration the quality of the patient's life after surgery.

We conducted pre-op diagnostic studies. Angiography showed us where the main blood vessels were and how they would be affected by the surgery. We determined that the femoral artery could be detached from the tumor, which allowed us to remove the mass and save her leg. Through our analyses, we found that the aggressive tumor was encapsulated. Thankfully there were no metastases. We detached the femoral artery from the tumor and successfully removed the large malignant mass. Then we reconstructed her leg. She recovered well from the surgery, and just a few days after, she was able to walk out of the hospital on her own power.

It was a complicated and delicate surgery. It was not merely removing the tumor. Care had to be taken to preserve each nerve, tendon, artery and vein. It was not easy to position the skin and stitch it together, for proper healing, after such a large tumor had been removed. The surgery took thirteen hours. Seeing the young woman walk again made it worth all of the painstaking effort. Five years later, she sent us a thank you card with a picture of her walking on the beach with her four-year-old son.

THE VALUE OF SURGICAL TRAINING

A lot of what I have been able to do as a surgeon can be attributed to the high-quality training I received at the University of Vienna's large teaching hospital in Vienna, Austria. I had to learn German at the same time as I was learning cancer surgery methods. As the instructors noticed that my German was minimal when I first enrolled, they placed me in the operating room rather than the classroom. I did many surgeries—about six hundred per year in my five-year residency. Over that period of performing approximately three thousand surgeries, I became quite fluent in oncology surgical methods and the German language too.

Learning traditional skills, in any discipline, is necessary before alternative and innovative techniques can be developed. Consider Pablo Picasso. He is widely revered as an artistic genius, though I find his abstract paintings to be, well, not very appealing. Let's just say that I prefer many drawings my children did while they were in pre-school. Before Picasso ventured into alternative abstract art, he was trained in classical art technique. He was gifted and could recreate

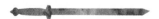

conventional, classic and realistic paintings. He only began abstract cubism after mastering traditional skills and conventions. He was a proficient painter, and once he had solidified his foundational skills, he had the potential to experiment and explore alternative approaches to art. Picasso changed it up on the art scene, and his cubism became an art revolution.

For us surgeons, quality formal training, like what I received in Vienna, gives us the foundation necessary to explore and develop new techniques. A unique philosophy is required to spark a medical revolution. My philosophy was formed on my father's teachings. He taught me first to, "Do no harm," and then to "Love my patient as I love myself," which boils down to Jesus' teachings to, "Do unto others as you would have others do unto you,"[18] and to, "Love your neighbor as yourself."[19]

To show how these principles are applied, take the example of a commando surgery. This surgery is used on patients with squamous-cell carcinomas of the head and neck, which can include tumors in the tongue, tonsils, gingiva, buccal mucosa and pharynx.[20]

A commando surgery typically involves the excision of a large portion of the neck and lower jaw. It's appalling to note that the procedure was named after military commandos trained to sneak up on enemies and slit throats in silence as a means to not alert the enemy to a covert operation. It is an aggressive surgery that is difficult to do. While I am capable of undertaking such an operation, I would not do it to my worst enemy. There is a fifty-five percent five-year survival rate after the surgery, but the negative impact on the quality of life outweighs the potential benefits.[21] Based on our principles, we would not recommend a commando surgery because of the long-term repercussions.

Practicing conservative surgery reflects our philosophy of focusing on the patient's quality of life above all.

The young mother whose leg we operated on, and saved, was an example of doing unto others as we would want them to do unto us. Though the standard of care would have been to remove the whole leg, which is a relatively easy surgery, we took on a complicated task to remove the tumor and reconstruct the leg to recover full functionality once again. Other surgeons would have cut off the leg. We didn't amputate because our philosophy is to do unto others what we would want to be done to us. Our medical philosophy has changed up surgery at Oasis of Hope.

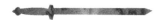

CHEMOTHERAPY

The most common treatment for cancer is chemotherapy. Chemotherapy doesn't discriminate. It is an equal opportunity destroyer of both malignant cells and healthy cells. It is so toxic that isolation rooms are used to prepare it, and the nurses that prepare it must wear protective equipment to not be harmed. Many chemotherapies provoke terrible side effects due to the toxicity. Common side effects include nausea, severe vomiting, uncontrollable diarrhea and hair loss. Sometimes, patients will suffer from kidney failure or liver failure due to chemotherapy.

Chemotherapy is an equal opportunity destroyer of cancerous cells and healthy cells.

Chemo drugs cause severe gastritis, which is another contributing factor to nausea. Chemo-associated gastritis is a severe irritation of the mucosa throughout the entire gastrointestinal (GI) tract. Irritation may be felt from the mouth through to the anus resulting in nausea and diarrhea. Because chemotherapy is immune-suppressive, patients are vulnerable to infections along the GI tract.

Hair loss results because chemotherapy destroys hair follicles. Incredibly uncomfortable dry mouth can occur because salivary glands are often part of the collateral damage of chemotherapy. Salivary glands are fast-growing cells, so they are usually affected first because chemo attacks fast-growing cells.

Another fast-growing organ affected by chemotherapy is bone marrow. Due to this, chemotherapy lowers the blood count, and anemia is a common negative side effect. Bone marrow is the primary lymphoid organ that generates lymphocytes. The attack on bone marrow explains why chemotherapy destroys the immune system. It attacks bone marrow, the blood cell factory, including the white cells that make up the immune system. A suppressed immune system increases the susceptibility to infections and promotes the progression of cancer. Have you ever wondered why chemotherapy is so toxic? Read on.

WORLD WAR I CHEMICAL WARFARE ROOTS

Chemotherapy was born out of the chemical warfare program in World War I. Scientists noted that soldiers exposed to mustard gas would experience bone marrow and lymph node depletion. Let us clarify, the USA never deployed mustard gas as it was determined to be too cruel. The observation happened after an accidental spill of sulfur mustard gas.[22] Seeing what

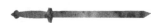

happened to the soldiers exposed to it, scientists at Yale University began experimenting with mustard gas to treat tumors in rats. You read right. The chemical weapon mustard gas became the first chemotherapy to treat cancer. Milton Winternitz was the lead cancer researcher at Yale in charge of the mustard gas experiments. He had also been the principal chemist working on mustard gas as a weapon in World War I.

The shift away from systemic chemotherapy would be revolutionary.

THE FAILURE OF CHEMOTHERAPY

Chemotherapy has significantly evolved since its weapon of mass destruction origin. Though it has become much more sophisticated, a comprehensive review of the five-year survival rates in twenty-two types of adult malignancies qualified chemotherapy as a complete failure. The data was collected from the USA's Surveillance Epidemiology and End Results (SEER) and Australia's cancer registry. The results are disheartening. The researchers wrote, "The overall contribution of curative and adjuvant cytotoxic chemotherapy to 5-year survival in adults was estimated to be 2.3% in Australia and 2.1% in the USA."[23] The fact that chemotherapy is such a small contributor to the five-year survival rate, in most cancers, makes it imperative for oncologists to change up when and how chemotherapy is used.

TARGETED DRUGS

Newer drugs, known as targeted drugs, have the potential to make systemic chemotherapy obsolete. The era of toxic chemotherapy, as we know it, could come to an end within the next five to ten years. The only cancers that respond well to chemotherapy are lymphomas and leukemia. The high-intensity chemotherapy regimens for these cancers achieve a seventy percent long-term survival rate.[24] A welcome change would be leaving toxic chemotherapies in the past. The paradigm shift away from systemic chemotherapy would be revolutionary in the field of medicine. We urge the oncology community to change up the use of chemotherapy.

Side effects and efficacy of targeted drugs are being studied. Though targeted therapies' mechanisms of action are much different than chemotherapy, many still produce severe side effects like nausea, vomiting and hair loss. Fortunately, researchers are addressing these issues. The drawback on targeted drugs is the cost. As explained in chapters two and nine, a single treatment can have a cost of $10,000.00 up to

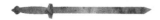

$475,000.00. Another downside is that they often are only effective for four to six months. We are hopeful that the costs will come down over time.

MANAGING SIDE EFFECTS

Alternative cancer treatments were born out of the need to minimize the adverse side effects associated with conventional oncology. Alternative medicine can help patients manage side effects while going through chemotherapy. Plant-based nutrition and supplements can increase a patient's tolerance of chemotherapy. Oncologists do not readily recommend dietary support for their patients because they do not understand the mechanism of action. It's not logical that oncologists don't dive into studying nutrition when many patients report positive benefits from eating healing foods. Indeed, there is no question that patients who partake in alternative medicine, exercise and eat a healthy diet, will better tolerate chemotherapy better than those who do not. Studies have shown that chemotherapy's response would improve when supplemented with exercise.[25] We have noticed that our results have improved due to exercise, vitamins, minerals and a healthy diet. Incorporating exercise and plant-based nutrition is foundational for all cancer patients, whether they come to Oasis of Hope or not.

AN ALTERNATIVE USE OF CHEMOTHERAPY

The way that chemotherapy is widely used is something we don't recommend. But, chemotherapy can be used in alternative manners to kill cancer cells without producing severe negative side effects. At Oasis of Hope, if we prescribe chemotherapy, we use the lowest effective dose.

Low-dose metronomic chemotherapy is effective and well-tolerated over an extended period.

All drugs have an effective dose range that can span hundreds of milligrams. What an effective dose range? Have you ever heard the phrase, "Take two aspirins and call me in the morning?" If a doctor always prescribes two aspirins, why don't drug makers simply make one bigger aspirin instead of two smaller ones? The answer is that the effective range of action to get rid of a headache is between one and two aspirins. Hence, the sensible thing to do is to take just one aspirin, and if the pain does not go away, then take the second one. Doctors prescribe two to avoid having a patient complain that a single aspirin didn't work. That may be ok for aspirin, but when it comes to chemotherapy, the higher the dose is, the more severe side effects will be.

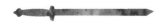

Chemotherapy has effective dose ranges, but oncologists tend to start with on the high end. However, there could be a big difference between the lower and higher limits of a chemotherapy's effective range. The Oasis of Hope changeup on chemotherapy is that we have learned that less is more. We always start on the lower end of the effective range, and then, if necessary, we slowly and gradually increase the dose until we find what works best for the individual patient. In this way, we don't provoke unbearable negative side effects by prescribing a higher dose than necessary. Low-dose chemotherapy can be effective and used over a long period.

There are several methods to administer low-dose chemotherapy. The main one that we use is a low-dose metronomic protocol. The word *metronomic* refers to having specific times when the drug is administered. Just as a metronome marks the time and rhythm of a song, low-dose chemotherapy given at specific times over a period. The low dose avoids adverse side effects. Dosing, spread out over time, can maintain a patient in the therapeutic range for a longer period. The extended period of use is what makes it effective.

Flooding the body with chemotherapy makes a patient suffer severe side effects. The therapeutic benefit of normal-dose is limited to the amount of time a patient can tolerate the therapy. In contrast, low-dose metronomic chemotherapy is highly tolerable, and increases the duration of therapeutic benefit. Clinical studies on low-dose metronomic chemotherapy conclude that it can induce disease control in advanced-stage cancer while lowering the adverse effects associated with standard doses of chemotherapy.[26] It is also proven to be quite effective when combined with COX-2 inhibitors, VEGF inhibitors, angiogenesis inhibitors and proapoptotic drugs. Studies such as these provide irrefutable evidence of our combination therapy approach.[27] The proapoptotic action of amygdalin contributes to the efficacy of our low-dose metronomic capecitabine protocol.

Combination therapies improve treatment outcomes.

We do not expect low-dose chemotherapy to work on its own. We combine it with natural and alternative therapies that enhance the activity of chemotherapy, or compliment it fighting the tumor. An integrative attack on the tumor is more effective than traditional chemotherapy. By combining alternative therapies with chemotherapy, we simply need less of the latter.

Combination therapies improve treatment outcomes. For example, studies show that radiation therapy is enhanced by

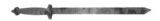

hyperthermia, and the patient will need less radiation. The two therapies compound or potentiate each other. In a previous chapter, we mentioned how hyperthermia enhances the effectiveness of HDIVC as well.

Prodrugs are a great change on chemotherapy.

PRODRUGS

Capecitabine, also known as Xeloda, is a prodrug alternative to chemotherapy. Scientists define a prodrug as, "A drug substance that is inactive in the intended pharmacological actions and is converted into the pharmacologically active agent by metabolic or physiochemical transformation."[28] Ok, cool. Wait, what does that mean?

Let's define a prodrug with clear language. A prodrug is a biologically inactive compound that is activated with metabolized by an organ or a tumor. When the body metabolizes the prodrug, a drug is produced. Capecitabine is a prodrug converted into the 5FU chemotherapy when metabolized in the liver or the tumors itself. The conversion to 5FU happens because an enzyme called cytidine deaminase that is highly concentrated in the liver and tumor tissues. Cytidine deaminase converts capecitabine into the compound 5′-DFUR. Various types of solid tumors have up to ten times the amounts of thymidine phosphorylase, which metabolizes 5′-DFUR into the active drug 5FU.[28]

Using capecitabine provides multiple advantages over the standard infusion of 5FU. The first is that it can be taken orally. The second is that it goes through the body, as a non-toxic substance, and becomes chemotherapy when it reaches the tumor. Because of those two factors, side effects are mild. Some of our patients don't have any side effects at all. The ones that do say that they are easily tolerated.

5FU was developed in the 1950s and has shown efficacy in adenocarcinomas, most specifically colorectal cancer. It is also extremely effective in clearing liver metastases. Its low toxicity rate makes it one of the best tolerated. For instance, 5-FU does not cause nausea and vomiting, unlike its peers, nor does it induce hair loss, except in very high doses.

Before capecitabine was available, we developed a surgical procedure to treat liver metastases locally with 5FU. We would place catheters directly into the liver to deliver the 5FU locally and effectively destroy metastases without side effects. In contrast, a systemic dose of 5FU to destroy liver metastases would need to be quite high, and the patient would suffer

adverse effects. Delivering 5FU locally was an elegant alternative, but then capecitabine was introduced. Now, we don't have to put the patient through surgery to deliver 5FU locally to liver metastases. Capecitabine goes directly to hepatic tumors, is converted to 5FU and gets excellent results for most patients. Prodrugs, like capecitabine, have provided a favorable changeup on chemotherapy.

OFF-LABEL DRUG USE

Another promising changeup in medicine is off-label drug use. When a drug is initially tested, the Food and Drug Administration (FDA) approval will be given only for the therapeutic benefit demonstrated during the initial trials. As the drug begins to be widely used, clinical observations are made. It's often discovered that a drug can be effective and safe for treating other ailments that were not tested in the initial clinical study presented to the FDA. Off-label drug use is a widely accepted practice because physicians' use is how clinical experience occurs. If a doctor notes that a dose different than the FDA approved recommended dose is more effective, prescribing that different dose qualifies as an off-label drug use. Using a drug for any therapeutic effect other than what the drug was initially approved for is off-label drug use.[27] Our use of

Metformin is the perfect example. It's a drug approved for diabetes management. But multiple clinical studies have demonstrated it as valid for cancer treatment because it selectively inhibits cancer stem cells.

Let us clarify an important fact. The FDA does not regulate physicians and medical practices. Therefore, there is nothing illegal about off-label drug use. Oasis of Hope is not alone in the off-label use of drugs like Metformin and capecitabine.

MD Anderson cancer treatment center has done studies on off-label use of capecitabine and published recommended doses that differ with the FDA guidelines.

In the case of capecitabine, though the FDA initially approved it for colorectal cancer, we have observed that it is effective in other solid tumors. We use it with most of our patients, because many studies confirm that off-label use of capecitabine works with multiple types of cancer. The MD Anderson study demonstrated that it is an effective therapy for metastatic breast cancer.[29] This is in line with our clinical experience. Again, off-label drug use is another great changeup on the way cancer treatment is done.

When it comes to oncology, there are many options of what, how and when to apply certain therapies, within permissible guidelines. It is strange how oncologists limit possibilities.

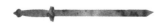

DO UNTO OTHERS

On a personal note, my father inspired me to change the way I would treat my patients. He provided a hands-on learning experience in which another doctor would lay hands on me and put me through a medical procedure that I had been performing on every patient. Here is how my father taught me to do unto others what I would want to be done unto me!

After I returned from my surgical training in Austria, I began modernizing our surgical department. In Vienna, I had trained extensively in endoscopy. I had become proficient at upper GI and lower GI endoscopy. Back in the early 1980s, we didn't have either colonoscopy or gastroscopy at Oasis of Hope, so I purchased both apparatuses. Patients started coming to us because we were among the first in Tijuana to provide endoscopic procedures. Soon, we began making proper diagnoses of colon carcinoma. For patients with colon carcinoma, it was a means for me to determine a tumor's status. A biopsy could be taken readily during a colonoscopy.

The trend of using colonoscopy as a screening tool was being developed. I got in front of the curve and began believing in its capabilities a little too much. Thus, I started doing colonoscopies very frequently. Everybody who would come to the hospital would get a colonoscopy. That was one of the first policies I established and imposed on all patients.

After a couple of months of doing hundreds of colonoscopies, my father called me to his office. He said, "Francisco, I noticed the other day that you are doing many colonoscopies." I replied, "Yes, you need to come and see. It's wonderful. You insert a tube, with a built-in camera, through the rectum. You can see inside the colon and find anything that is wrong."

While I was explaining this "exciting" technology to my father, he started writing a prescription. I thought that my father was not interested in what I was explaining, so I asked, "What are you writing?" He replied, "A prescription for a colonoscopy." I was taken aback and asked, "A colonoscopy? For whom?" He looked up at me and answered, "For you, Francisco." Hence, I had to get somebody else to do my colonoscopy, and since there were not too many people trained in colonoscopy, I had a hard time finding someone. Fortunately, I had a friend who did it for me. Thus, I had my first eve colonoscopy. This experience was eye-opening for me. It was not fun whatsoever.

I learned what it felt like to have a three-foot-long tube inserted into my rectum to insufflate the colon, explore and evaluate. After that, you have to wash it out with fluids. Of

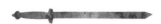

course, my father did not make me go through the procedure as some sort of punishment. There was a fundamental lesson here. I experienced exactly what a patient goes through with the procedures we do. It was a perfect and unforgettable lesson for me. I am not saying a colonoscopy is not as effective as I thought it was, because it is undoubtedly a great tool. The point is that a procedure should only be used on patients when it is necessary. Far too often, we doctors overuse procedures just because they are there for us to use. My father helped me learn that lesson quite well.

My father had me undergo a colonoscopy to help increase my empathy for patients I was performing the procedure on.

My father was strictly doing oncology at the time. He always chose to remain focused on the task at hand. He was the one who developed the philosophy to not over-prescribe, not be too aggressive, take a step at a time and preserve the quality of a patient's life above all. This methodology may seem obvious, but many physicians get swept up with the advances in medicine, and medical devices, and forget about the patient's well being and treatment experience. My father taught me always to remain faithful to my medical ideals and care for patients to the best of my ability. He taught me to go above and beyond what is expected.

OASIS OF HOPE ONE-TWO-THREE-PUNCH

One of the most potent Oasis of Hope changeups on cancer is how we modulate therapies. Our approach is similar to Nolan Ryan's pitching. We throw a fastball followed by a curveball and then an off-speed pitch. The batter (cancer) never knows what's coming. We might even throw a beanball to hit the batter intentionally. We call our changeup strategy the *One-Two-Three-Punch*. It's like a boxer that delivers a body blow followed by a hook to the jaw, and hopefully, the third punch will knock cancer out. The opponent never learns how to defend himself because he never knows what is coming next.

Our One-Two-Three-Punch strategy aims to prevent cancer from developing resistance to treatment.

For nearly six decades, we have been refining this strategy because cancer cells are incredibly resilient and capable of developing resistance against treatments. The threat of recurrence is ever-present when cancer is only treated with aggressive therapies such as chemotherapy and radiation. Our

one-two-three-punch aims to prevent cancer from developing resistance to a specific treatment. We keep cancer off balance by modulating oxidative therapies with antioxidative therapies.

Oxidative treatments such as chemotherapy, radiation, and even our natural HDIVC, are effective at knocking down cancer. But, our second punch is made up of treatments that include antioxidants. The home therapy we prescribe to our patients is usually an antioxidant regimen. When patients come back for a follow-up booster treatment, we hit cancer with a third punch of oxidative therapies. Then we re-evaluate and make whatever changes needed to keep cancer from regaining its balance. Changing treatment up makes it difficult for cancer to gain the necessary momentum for a full recurrence.

Our changeup strategy frequently helps a patient outlive the original prognosis given by an oncologist before coming to Oasis of Hope. The one-two-three punch strategy is vital, even with alternative cancer therapies, because of cancer's ability to mutate and develop resistance against any type of therapy.

WE ARE HOLISTIC

Another valuable changeup we have done in cancer care is providing wrap-around body, mind and spirit treatment. Current oncology protocols are developed with a reductionist mentality. The search for a single cancer-killing molecule is the focus of cancer drug development. The goal of pharmaceutical companies is to produce specialized chemotherapies that target a specific type of tumor. Another reductionist strategy is to target one specific oncogene by a drug or virus. In sharp contrast, the Oasis of Hope approach is holistic.

Oasis of Hope's commitment to holism versus reductionism is apparent when you meet and receive treatment from our multidisciplinary team.

In humans, a single molecule cannot explain any one function in the body. Each function requires a multitude of proteins, enzymes, nutrients and elements to interact. Our combination therapies work on many different levels in the attack against cancer. Cancer has several metabolic traits that we can exploit with various treatments that undermine cancer's strongholds. At any given point, we may employ as many as twenty different cancer-fighting agents in our protocols.

A reductionist oncology program is hyper-specialized. Patients only oncologists who would only deal with cancer. Oasis of Hope considers the total health of a patient.

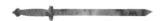

For by wise counsel you will wage your war, and in multitude of counselors there is safety.
—Proverbs 24:6 MEV

THE OASIS OF HOPE MULTIDISCIPLINARY TEAM

At traditional oncology centers, a patient doesn't receive the benefit of seeing doctors and health practitioners from various specialties. But, patients need to see more than an oncologist because anyone who has cancer will have some non-cancer-related health issues as well. We don't look at our patients through an oncologist's lens only. We have put together an outstanding group of specialists that can provide perspectives from different angles. The Oasis of Hope multidisciplinary team is comprised of a clinical oncologist, surgical oncologists, hematologist, internist, psychosocial oncology physician, radiologist, family medicine specialist, nutritionists, psychologist, spiritual counselor and researchers. We put this multitude of counselors to work for each patient combating cancer.

Each week, our multidisciplinary team meets for hours to go through every patient's case. Each expert makes observations from what they see through the lens of their specialty. In this way, we provide an advantage for our patients that other oncology centers cannot offer. Our oncologist monitors a tumor's evolution and response to our natural therapies. They can advise on potential benefits of low-dose chemotherapy or radiation. Our surgical oncologists evaluate and look for any advantage of debulking a tumor, doing a biopsy, clearing out any bowel obstruction, facilitating intratumoral treatments or other surgical procedures. Our hematologist addresses abnormalities in the blood, assesses damage to the bone marrow from chemotherapy or radiation, measures immunity and coordinates immunotherapies. Our internist monitors each organ's function, oversees hyperthermia, and does procedures such as catheter installations or draining lungs or the peritoneum. Our medical doctor, trained in palliative care and psychosocial oncology, evaluates a patient's emotional distress. She provides counsel and interventions to help a patient cope. Our radiologist interprets imaging studies and provides insight. The radiologist helps us evaluate the patient's evolution by comparing scans done before the patient started treatment at Oasis of Hope with scans done after our therapies. Our family medicine specialist addresses primary care health issues. Our nutritionists coordinate food and juice regimens, and develop protocols for patients with specific dietary. Our psychologist provides group and individual counseling to teach coping techniques and facilitate emotional healing. Our pastor provides spiritual support through daily devotions and prayer for all patients open to prayer. Our researchers keep us up to date on the latest findings, and measure the changes in our patients' conditions and outcomes. They provide us the data we need to make improvements. All of these different practitioners work in concert for the benefit of our patients. Having a multidisciplinary team is key to our ability to change things up as needed to undermine cancer.

We treat the patient, not the disease.

PATIENT-CENTERED

Our founder, Dr. Ernesto Contreras, Sr. said, "We're not treating the tumor, we are treating the patient." This treatment principle drives our goal of improving the quality of life of our patients. Because we are patient-centered rather than tumor-focused, we look beyond cancer to evaluate a patient's overall wellness. A health concern, entirely not related to cancer, may be making a patient's life miserable. Imagine if the patient has an ingrown toenail and can't walk. Because it's not cancer-related, an oncologist will likely not address it. At Oasis of Hope, we will resolve the ingrown toenail for the patient, because we are patient-focused and know that it is a quality of life issue.

Dr. Contreras, Sr. realized the importance of this. He taught us that our pursuit should not be eradicating cancer; it should be extending life and improving the quality of life our patients enjoy. Correcting health issues affecting a patient's quality of life, though not directly related to cancer, will provide a patient with great relief and free up energy to fight cancer better.

Being patient-centered is a compassionate changeup in cancer treatment.

DON'T ASSUME IT'S THE CANCER

Being patient-centered helps us be aware of everything a patient may be experiencing. It also allows us to help our patients deal with fears. Patients frequently assume that every little pain indicates that cancer is getting worse. If a patient suddenly has an aching joint in the knee, they instantly worry, "Oh my God, cancer has spread to my knee." The possibility that arthritis may be developing after a life of playing tennis, or that there may be a strain or a sprain, doesn't cross their mind. Cancer produces quite a bit of fear, so it is easy to jump to

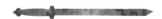

conclusions that everything negative change in health is being caused by cancer. We examine a patient whenever a new health problem presents to clarify that not every ache, pain or illness is related to the disease.

ALL UNDER ONE ROOF

By having a multidisciplinary team, we can address, and often resolve, side health issues. Also, we don't have to refer patients out to get emotional support, nutritional support, education and classes. We meet most of a patient's need right at the hospital. Anxiety is lower when a patient doesn't have to coordinate multiple consultations with different specialists in different locations.

The theme of this chapter is to change things up. We don't only change things up on cancer. We also change up the scope of treatments we provide. We address what oncologists may consider being secondary and tertiary health issues. It isn't uncommon for an oncologist to dismiss non-cancer-related issues and to advise patients to forget about other problems because they need to take care of cancer above all. It's wrong to dismiss any health issue that diminishes a patient's quality of life, and this dismissive attitude of oncologists adds to the feeling of gloom and doom patients often experience at typical oncology centers.

THE SMILE PHENOMENA

A few years back, we had the opportunity to be given a tour of the most prominent integrative cancer treatment centers whose advertising budget is so large they have had *Super Bowl* ads. We share this story not as a criticism, but as an illustration of how Oasis of Hope is different. That massive oncology treatment system has multiple hospitals built with hundreds of millions of dollars. We were excited to learn something new. We were deflated when we observed the patients in treatment. Though their marketing message made their hospital look like the patient experience would be extraordinary, it was the same as other ordinary oncology centers we had visited. Patients were isolated, and there were no smiles. We started the tour on the first floor and waited at an elevator. When the doors opened, we were saddened to see a patient in a wheelchair with a small trashcan attached to the side. She needed it as she was vomiting due to the chemotherapy she had just received. Do you know what was painfully missing at that center? Smiles.

At Oasis of Hope, we've changed up the typical cancer treatment process to an extraordinary healing experience. We

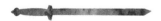

have a community treatment room where patients can visit with each other while receiving treatment. We provide education, group counseling and worship times in the community treatment room. Meals are served in the dining commons, where we have round tables so patients can share meals and fellowship. No one is isolated. A community of support is felt at Oasis of Hope. Our hospital a community of hope. We also have movie nights, bingo and other activities that promote friendship, fellowship and joy. What is the result of our changeup to the typical cancer treatment experience? You will see more smiles on the faces of our patients, companions and staff faces than in any other oncology center in the world.

SMILES = QUALITY OF LIFE

CONCLUSION

We began this chapter with Sun Tzu's quote that states that knowing how to vary military tactics gives a general a significant advantage. We refer to the varying of tactics as a changeup. Here is how Oasis of Hope has changed up the traditional cancer treatment model:

- We care for the whole patient—body, mind and spirit.
- We share the healing power of faith, hope and love.
- We advance medical science to put an end to cancer, one patient at a time.

- We are patient-centered, not disease-focused.
- We focus on the quality of life, not tumor eradication.
- We practice conservative organ-preserving surgeries.
- We provide oxygen therapy for patients undergoing radiotherapy.
- We administer low-dose metronomic chemotherapy.
- We prescribe whole food plant-based nutrition and exercise to promote the immune system and decrease negative side effects.
- We use prodrugs as alternatives to chemotherapy.
- We employ evidence-based off-label drug use.
- We treat our patients as we would want to be treated.
- We modulate oxidative therapies with anti-oxidative therapies to keep cancer from developing resistance.
- We are holistic, not reductionists.
- We fortify the spirit and care for the soul to promote healing in the body.
- Our multidisciplinary team looks after the overall health of our patients, including emotional and spiritual health.
- We have multiple services, such as oncology, nutrition and counseling, all under one roof.
- We empower patients through education.
- We champion a patient's right to choose treatments.
- Prayer is the first line of defense, not the last resort.

It is striking how peaceful it is at Oasis of Hope. You could not imagine everything that goes into providing the healing experience that benefits our patients in ways that conventional cancer centers cannot. Many people work tirelessly behind the scenes to provide and incredible Oasis of Hope healing experience. There is one motivating factor behind everything we do. It is you. Our reason to exist is you.

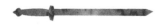

STORY OF HOPE

Kristen James • Triple Negative Breast Cancer • 2015

In January 2015, I was diagnosed with triple-negative breast cancer. I talked to many doctors and felt as if there was no hope. That's when I found the book *Beating Cancer* by Dr. Contreras. After reading the book in one night, followed by much prayer, I felt like Oasis of Hope was the path God had for me. I chose to have no treatments in the US, and I headed straight for Tijuana. I had surgery to remove my tumor, which they used to program my dendritic cell vaccine. Then I went through the scheduled treatments at Oasis of Hope.

The environment was very spiritual and uplifting. The staff was friendly and always willing to answer questions. I talked with other patients, listened to their stories and found encouragement in returning patients' stories. We all supported and encouraged each other as we were all in this together. We would have treatments in the morning and often take walks on the beach together in the afternoon.

I left Oasis of Hope cancer-free and am still in complete remission. I have made friends that I will remember forever. People often call and ask about my experience and if I would make the same choice again. My answer is always 100% yes. I am so glad that God provided me with Dr. Contreras' book, which led me to Mexico. I can never thank Dr. Contreras and his staff enough for all they have done for me.

—Kristen James
Winston Salem, North Carolina
USA

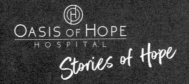

STORY OF HOPE

Jim Barry • Prostate Cancer • 2015

I was diagnosed with prostate cancer, adenocarcinoma tumor, in October of 2015. The urologist, here in Cody, recommended surgery after doing tests and biopsies. I didn't think highly of the recommendation. I started researching on my own and getting information from cancer patients. I knew two people treated by Oasis of Hope. They were delighted with the treatment and had come away with excellent results. I started leaning toward that.

Another cancer patient that had been at Oasis of Hope asked me, "What does it take for me to convince you to go to the hospital for treatment?" That's what led me to Oasis of Hope. When I found out that it was a Christian-based ministry, I told my wife that I would be going to Oasis of Hope for treatment. We started making travel plans.

They provide treatments for the body, like the vaccine, hyperthermia, and the other therapies given in combination to fight cancer. But they treat the whole person–body, mind, and soul. The emotional treatment gives hope that treatment will help and that things are going to be okay. The diet, emotional support and spiritual treatment, combined with the physical treatment, make the treatment so much different from many other places. If you go to many hospitals in the States, they'll do physical treatments, whether surgery, chemo or radiation, but there's a lack of emotional support for a person, whereas Oasis of Hope addresses that.

It's become what I call "my treatment family." The atmosphere facilitates that with a family-style dining area where you sit around with other patients and staff and converse about hope and treatments. You can openly talk about cancer, and other things too. It's very encouraging and brightens things up when you visit daily with other patients that have had successful treatments. Then the worship times in the morning were a real big thing for me. That really made my days, and just gave me a lot of hope, and refocused my mind on something other than on the disease. It helped me stop worrying so much about cancer. It helped me a lot.

I'm doing well now. I've had two PET scans and two MRIs that show no activity of cancer. I'm very thankful. Praise the Lord for that. I'm thankful and blessed for that. I'm very grateful for the treatment that I've received from the hospital and think very highly of the nurses, the doctors, and the staff. I look forward to going back again for a checkup and seeing my treatment family again.

—Jim Barry
Cody, Wyoming
United States

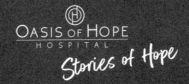

行軍

ELEVEN

MOBILIZE

If you are careful of your soldiers, this will spell victory.
—Sun Tzu
The Art of War
The Army on the March

O z, the land at the end of the *Yellow Brick Road*, held the promise of returning Dorothy home, giving the Tin Woodman a heart, the Scarecrow a brain and the Lion courage.[1] The golden pathway was exciting and enticing, but of course, it was full of challenges. Dorothy and Toto joined their new friends on the venture that would take them through the *Dark Forest*, where they would certainly encounter lions and tigers and bears, oh my!

Under the leadership of the ruby-slippered heroine, this little army had to mobilize to march into the darkness. Every tree in the mysterious forest could be obscuring multiple threats. The comrades were unsure of which way to go. They did not know if they had the *heart* to move forward, the *brains* to overcome obstacles or the *courage* to march in the face of fear.

The perilous forest trek revealed that each person already possessed what they thought was missing. Dorothy found that home is where the heart is. The Tin Woodman's unfailing loyalty to Dorothy revealed that he had a heart. The Scarecrow learned so much along the way, which showed that he had a brain because it takes brains to learn! Later, he was named the wisest man in Oz. The cowardly lion thought that courage was the absence of fear. But courage is marching forward in the face of fear. He showed immense courage when he held off the *Kalidah* monsters in the forest so the Tin Woodman could cut down a tree and make a bridge to escape over a ravine. The team of misfits was successful because they mobilized despite the challenges that laid before them.

The Psalmist pointed to the ultimate source of strength to march through the enemy's territory declaring:

Even though I walk through the valley of the shadow of death, I will fear no evil; for You are with me; Your rod and Your staff, they comfort me.[2]
—Psalm 23:4

No matter the threat, you must mobilize your troops if you are to overcome the challenge.

You may be asking, "What troops? I don't have any troops." News flash, you do! You have a mighty military force living inside you fighting every millisecond of the day for you.

Your immune system is the fiercest cancer-fighting force on earth.

YOUR MILITARY MIGHT

Your incredible endogenous armed forces are your God-given defenses—the immune system. The immune system is the most potent and effective anticancer agent known to humankind. When it is working perfectly, the probability of a tumor forming is nearly zero. In most cases, patients taking chemotherapy, or radiation, to fight cancer have a diminished immune system. Conventional therapies severely damage immune cells. We provide therapies to nurture and restore your natural defenses. It's an important therapeutic objective because each cell that makes up part of your immune system is a soldier that will go to battle for you.

The master military strategist Sun Tzu knew that it was critical to take care of his soldiers. He said, "If you are careful of

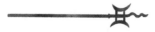

your men, and camp on hard ground, the army will be free from disease of every kind, and this will spell victory."[3]

Your immune system is truly a force to be reckoned with.

HOW YOUR IMMUNE SYSTEM WORKS

Your immune system is the military might that defends your body against pathogens that can cause infections and disease— including cancer.[4] Pathogens are foreign bodies such as viruses, bacteria, and microorganisms.[5]

The parts of the immune system:

- Skin is the exterior barrier and first line of defense.
- Cilia line the respiratory tract and work to expel foreign bodies.
- Hydrochloric acid, produced by the stomach, destroys microorganisms.
- Intestinal flora inhibits the growth of pathogens.
- Lymph nodes secrete lymph to remove and expel pathogens from the body.
- White blood cells, produced within the bone marrow, seek, destroy and dissolve pathogens, infection and disease.

The immune system is well equipped with anticancer lymphocytes (white blood cells), including T lymphocytes (T cells)[6] and natural killer cells (NK cells). NK cells have enzymes that kill cancer cells and viruses.[7]

IMMUNE STRESSORS

The immune system can break down when a person is exposed to physical or emotional stressors. Examples of physical stressors include environmental toxins, such as pesticides and household cleansers, chronic infections, chemotherapy and radiation. Emotional stressors may include prolonged grieving, chronic fear or anxiety, relational problems and anything that promotes feelings of fear, anger, hurt, loss or resentment.

The immune response to stressors and pathogens is inflammation. Chronic inflammation is detrimental to the body, so the immune system produces Regulatory T cells (T reg cells) to suppress the immune response and keep it in check.[8] It is common for a patient's immune system to no longer be able to combat cancer due to T reg cell suppression. The immune system may be rendered unable to fight cancer by the damage that is done by chemotherapy and radiotherapy too.

CANCER'S DEFENSE MECHANISM

One reason why cancer is difficult to defeat is metabolic traits that form part of its defense mechanisms. A tumor's

microenvironment is capable of suppressing the anticancer immune response.

**A tumor's microenvironment suppresses
the body's anticancer immune response.**

Herein lies a challenge—how can an anticancer immune response be solicited when the tumor's microenvironment, and other factors such as chemotherapy, is suppressing the immune system? We answer that important question with a therapy that can undermine cancer's microenvironmental stronghold. We have developed a vaccine that targets cancer by encoding dendritic cells with a tumor-specific cancer antigen. We activate the patient's T cells and NK cells. We use the encoded dendritic cells to target the tumor for the activated attack.

A CANCER VACCINE: THE MEDICAL HOLY GRAIL

The polio vaccine has been effective in combating, and nearly eradicating, the poliovirus. In 2018, only eight cases of polio were reported.[10] Vaccines have been incredibly effective against many diseases. The *Medical Holy Grail* would be a vaccine that could eradicate cancer from the world.

A vaccine is defined as "Any preparation used as a preventive inoculation to confer immunity against a specific disease, usually employing an innocuous form of the disease agent, as killed or weakened bacteria or viruses, to stimulate antibody production."[11] Traditionally, vaccines are protective and given to a person to prevent the contraction of a specific illness. To date, there are protective vaccines for only two types of cancer—cervical cancer and liver cancer. These vaccines do not directly target cancer. Gardasil® and Cervarix® are vaccines designed to protect against strands of the human papillomavirus (HPV), which can cause cervical cancer.[12] The efficacy of these vaccines is debatable. More data is required to determine whether the immune response against HPV is translating to a decrease in cervical cancer. The liver cancer vaccine also does not target cancer. Instead, it targets the hepatitis B virus, which is associated with the development of liver cancer.[13]

Until recently, cancer vaccines are used for disease prevention, not treatment. There is a relatively new breakthrough in the preparation of a vaccine that can be used in the treatment of cancer. The National Cancer Institute describes this type of vaccine as "A substance or group of substances meant to cause the immune system to respond to a tumor or to microorganisms, such as bacteria or viruses. A

vaccine can help the body recognize and destroy cancer cells or microorganisms."[14]

DENDRITIC CELL VACCINE

A therapeutic vaccine is designed to administer to people who already have cancer. Its purpose is to induce an immune response capable of targeting specific cancer cells, killing them, slowing or reversing tumor growth, inhibiting metastases, and ultimately increasing survival rates.[15] This type of immunotherapy vaccine is categorized as a dendritic cell vaccine (DCV),[16] which is an antigen-presenting cell vaccine.[17] The efficacy and safety of DCVs have been demonstrated in multiple clinical trials in vitro, and in vivo with animals and humans. If fact, the FDA approved the first DCV in 2010 after phase three studies in patients with metastatic prostate cancer showed a three-year survival rate of thirty-four percent versus eleven percent.[18]

Before we explain how DCVs work, let us tell you what a dendritic cell (DC) is. A DC is an "antigen-presenting cell."[19] DCs have the capability of uptaking antigens cancer cells. Antigens are key to inducing an immune response.[20] Cancer cells produce antigens, which are tumor-specific proteins that reside on the surface of malignant cells. Antigens also circulate in the blood. Each tumor-specific antigen (TSA) is unique. Pathologists and oncologists are able to measure tumor activity in some cancers by using antigen counts as tumor markers. You are probably familiar with the term "PSA" because it is the most common test to screen for prostate cancer. PSA stands for prostate-specific antigen.[21] To clarify, antigens are not only specific to a cancer type, but they are also unique to the specific tumor in a patient. No two patients will have identical TSAs, even if they have the same diagnosis.

The tumor-destroying action of the immune system is elegant.

HOW A DCV WORKS

Dendritic cells (DCs) are used in vaccines because they specialize in capturing TSAs. Once a DC captures a TSA, it converts it from a protein into peptides that will attract T cells and NK cells.[22,23] In this way, DCs induce an immune response that will kill tumor cells. DCs also retain a memory of this

response, and if the TSA is detected in the future, it will induce a cancer-killing immune response again.[24,25]

It is remarkable how the various immune cells interact to destroy cancer. Think of a heat-seeking missile that is sent out to destroy a jet fighter. The infrared light emission given off by the jet engines would be the antigen. The DC would be the sensor that detects the infrared emission, targets it, and then guides the missile to the heat source. The T cells and NK cells would be the missile's explosive devices that would destroy the enemy jet fighter. This simple analogy illustrates the sophisticated and elegant tumor-destroying function of the immune system.

To summarize why DCs are at the center of cancer vaccine development, they can present T cells and NK cells to tumor cells. Once they are encoded with a TSA, they retain a memory of the transaction. The DC's memory makes it protective against the recurrence of tumors.

HOW WE PREPARE YOUR PERSONAL DCV

Cancerous cells circulate in the blood. As previously stated, malignant cells have antigens on their surfaces called "tumor-specific antigens." (TSA)[26] We collect TSAs through a blood draw. In some cases, the tumor is accessible, and we take a tissue sample, which is a rich source of TSAs. DC precursor cells are contained in the blood or tissue sample. They are cultivated and matured with cytokines such as Interleukin 4 (IL-4),[27] which will activate the T cells, and IL-15 to activate the NK cells.[28] The T cells that are stimulated in a laboratory to kill tumor cells are referred to as lymphokine-activated killer cells, or T-LAK cells. It is interesting to note that NK cells help DCs mature.[29] The TSA is used to pulse the DC and activate it.

There are numerous cultivation methods used to isolate TSAs from the blood or tissue samples. One involves repeatedly freezing and thawing the cells. Necrosis (cell destruction) is mimicked, and the TSA is isolated. Another method is to expose tumor cells to UV light, or gamma irradiation, which will mimic apoptosis (cell death) and isolate the TSA. Another method is to oxidize the tumor cells with hypochlorous acid (HOCL), which will provoke rapid necrosis.[30]

Once the DCs are encoded with the TSA, they are cultured and activated along with the T-LAK cells and NK cells. The vaccine is then ready for injection into the same patient who provided the TSA and immune cells. The T-LAK and activated NK cells are given back to the patient via infusions. Generally,

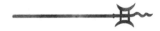

the vaccine is given in a series of injections and infusions with periods in between shots. The rest period provides time for the DCs, T-LAK cells, and NK cells to further mature and multiply in strength and numbers because the vaccine is made up of live cells.

AN ABUNDANCE OF SCIENTIFIC EVIDENCE

DCVs are being studied in vitro with cancer cell lines, and in vivo in animals and human patients. Results are being published from clinical trials conducted around the world. There is a preponderance of scientific evidence that DCVs are safe and effective. Let's take a look at a few peer-reviewed publications.

A clinical trial in Korea was conducted with breast cancer patients and kidney cancer patients. All patients tolerated the vaccine well. NK activity was induced in sixty percent of the patients.[31] Another clinical trial in China administered DCV to colorectal cancer patients. The DCV extended the disease-free period and generated longer survival rates. There was an increased cytotoxic (cancer cell destructive) response observed in fifty-seven percent of the patients.[32]

A study conducted with one hundred colorectal cancer patients demonstrated that more than seventy percent of the patients experienced an improvement in strength, sleep, appetite and weight. Thirty-three percent of the patients experienced adverse effects, including fever, loss of appetite, joint pain and skin rash. The side effects were mild, and the vaccine was well tolerated.[33] Another study conducted in China showed that DCVs have anti-tumor effects on bladder cancer cells.[34]

A group of researchers in Israel tested a DCV on patients with myeloma. They observed that the disease stopped progressing in sixty-six percent of the patients from several months up to two years after vaccination.[35]

DCVS OFFER HOPE

Let us bring to your attention three very encouraging clinical trials. The studies were conducted with patients presenting pancreatic cancer, lung cancer and metastatic melanoma. These cancer types have low five-year survival rates, so the clinical trial was crucial. The stage IV five-year survival rate for pancreatic cancer is two percent, lung cancer is under two percent, and melanoma is fifteen percent.[36]

Let us start with pancreatic cancer. It was a large study using data from seven treatment centers in Japan. It included two hundred and fifty-five patients with inoperable pancreatic cancer. The multi-center study concluded that DCVs were well tolerated, adverse reactions were mild, and they may improve outcomes in patients who are concurrently receiving chemotherapy or radiotherapy.[37]

A study on lung cancer was interesting because lung cancer is not generally considered immune-sensitive. The patients had non-small cell lung cancer. Some patients received the DCV, and the control group did not. The patients receiving DCV, showed a potent immune response.[38]

The trial with metastatic melanoma was conducted in the United Kingdom. All of the patients tolerated the vaccine well. Most of the patients experienced mild adverse effects, including skin irritation at the injection, site and flu-like symptoms. All of the patients experienced a good immune response. There was measurable tumor reduction in twelve percent of the patients, and tumor stabilization in sixteen percent of the patients.[39]

A clinical trial conducted in Lithuania included patients with prostate, kidney, and bladder cancer. There was an improved immune response in seventy percent of the patients and partial or complete remission in twenty percent of the patients.[40] This study, like the others, make a strong case that DCVs are essential in the treatment of cancer. Still, Oasis of Hope is one of the few centers in the world actively using DCV with its patients.

Some studies have shown how to enhance results of DCVs with other treatment protocols. There was a study conducted by Baylor Research Institute that concluded that the use of mild chemotherapies, such as cyclophosphamide (Cytoxan®), can suppress T reg cells before injecting the DCV resulting in a much more potent anticancer immune response.[41]

CYCLOPHOSPHAMIDE

Cyclophosphamide is a chemotherapy proven to target and destroy T reg cells specifically. Targeting T reg cells is effective because their levels are higher than normal in cancer patients.

If a patient has a high level of immune-suppressing T reg cells, we can lower the count with a low-dose IV of cyclophosphamide. Fortunately, our patients experience mild

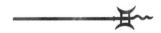

to no side effects. Not all of our patients have high levels of T reg cells. For those who have normal levels, we prescribe oral cyclophosphamide, which is even easier to tolerate, while still suppressing T reg cells.

LET'S NOT SPIN OUR WHEELS

What is the advantage of destroying T reg cells? Although our DCV elicits a great anticancer immune response, T reg cells work to suppress it. It's like having a souped-up Iacocca Limited-Edition 45th Anniversary Mustang, with 700 horsepower, and putting the pedal to the metal while mashing on the brakes. You'll have all the power in the world, but your wheels will spin and smoke until you release the breaks. The DCV is like a souped-up immune therapy, and T regs are the brakes. A little dose of cyclophosphamide will deactivate the breaks, and we are off to the races.

We want to clarify that T reg cells are not detrimental to our health. They are a vital part of our immune system because they modulate it and protect against autoimmune diseases like arthritis, Crohn's disease and asthma. So we need T reg cells, but we don't want them to act like the high-capacity brakes used in sports cars when it comes to cancer. By lowering the T reg cell count, the immune system is not suppressed and can combat cancer better.

CONCLUSION

Oasis of Hope has been developing and improving immunotherapies over the last six decades. In the past, we conducted a study using allogeneic immunotherapies. Cells were donated from a person to a patient. That was quite successful and emotional because Oasis of Hope team members stepped up and donated blood to meet our patients' needs. Our staff members were donating their cells to provide therapy for our patients. Patients were overwhelmed with gratitude and could thank the donor personally. The results were promising, but our DCV is superior to the allogeneic vaccine by far.

Our DCV is autologous immunotherapy. Autologous means it originates from the patient. The immune cells are harvested from the patient, cultured, and then infused or injected back into the patient. Autologous immunotherapy is much more effective than allogeneic immunotherapy. The patient's TSAs, DCs, T cells and NK cells are used. No therapy is more personalized than our DCV. The patient's DCs are encoded with the TSA harvested from the tumor or circulating cancer cells. The DC presents the tumor to the patient's matured T cells and

NK cells to do what they are designed to do—seek and destroy cancer. We don't consider the DCV a stand-alone therapy. It is an enhancement to our *Core* Oasis of Hope therapy. It is an excellent adjuvant therapy because it is effective at inducing an anticancer immune response, and in many cases, measurable reduction in the size of the tumor. From all of the clinical trials on DCVs being conducted at centers, it is reported that DCVs:

- Target malignant cells[42]
- Activate anti-tumor immunity[43]
- Induce anti-tumor cytotoxic T lymphocyte activity[44]
- Inhibit metastases[45]

We are encouraged by these studies because they confirm our experience and clinical observations with DCVs at Oasis of Hope. Numerous studies provide additional data for us to continuously advance our fight against cancer, which is essential because, at our core, Oasis of Hope practices patient-centered data-driven medicine.

We are confident that new clinical trials will show ways to further improve outcomes with DCVs. These studies will lead to breakthroughs in DCV development, and we are ready. Our DCV is effective. We plan to increase its potency by continuing research, implementing new methods to suppress T reg cells, and finding better methods to activate NK cells. One new intervention we are considering is harvesting TSAs from a tumor's fibroblasts (connective tissue).[46]

Research suggests that utilizing pharmaceuticals, such as colchicine, during the culturing of the DC may enhance its efficacy.[47] Phytochemicals, such as shikonin, may also enhance tumor immunogenicity of DCVs, as well.[48]

As we review results from each new clinical trial published every year, we double down on our research efforts and leverage our immunohematology laboratory. We benefit from the knowledge and experience of our oncologists, hematologists and dedicated researchers. We believe that our DCV is, and will continue to be one of the most effective cancer vaccines in the world.

Oasis of Hope practices patient-centered, data-driven medicine.

We are please to provide our potent and personalized Dendritic Cell Vaccine to all of our patients taking an Oasis of Hope *Enhanced* cancer treatment protocol.

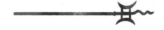

STORY OF HOPE

Susan Novak • Breast Cancer HR+ • 2003

The diagnosis of a five-centimeter tumor, that was an intermediate stage hormone receptive breast cancer, came to me as such a shock. I was a woman in her 50's with no history of cancer in the family. The tumor was removed at my local hospital in Soldotna, Alaska. The surgeon stated she "didn't get it all," but felt that it would be good enough because she didn't think it was cancer. The biopsy proved her wrong, and it was indeed, cancer. I knew of several success stories at Oasis of Hope Hospital, through my father-in-law. I wanted to try Oasis of Hope first before trying anything else.

The treatment was successful, and I began to see signs of tumor shrinkage even before I left Oasis of Hope. The improvements continued at home until all my tests showed no sign of cancer. I enjoyed a total recovery and resumed a normal lifestyle.

In 2010, I was diagnosed with recurrent breast cancer. A smaller tumor was removed, along with about four or five lymph nodes. I returned to Oasis of Hope for treatment. Once again, after treatment, I am cancer-free for ten years and enjoying good health and the everyday active lifestyle of a woman who is now 70!

Oasis of Hope changed my life. I have remained cancer-free and healthy, and through education at the hospital, I am more aware of how to eat well to maintain my health. I've also learned what supplements work best to fight cancer. The treatments build up your body and immune system instead of destroying it. It is a novel idea to much of western medicine. What a concept! I also made that body-mind-spirit connection, often mentioned at Oasis of Hope, embracing my faith as part of my recovery and learning how my emotions are tied to my health.

Oasis of Hope's proactive approach arms you with the knowledge you need to be successful: solid science and research explained well during the lectures; a professional and compassionate staff; cooking classes; good food; and great music and messages. And I must say, Dr. Contreras is a genius and an amazing doctor with the love of God in him! And Dr. Ceceña is a very wise and caring doctor who works tirelessly for his patients.

—Susan Novak
Kasilof, Alaska
United States

Addendum: In 2017, my husband was diagnosed with stage 3B colorectal cancer. He went to Oasis of Hope, of course. In June 2020, his MRI shows he continues to have no metastasis. No tumor can be found to measure!

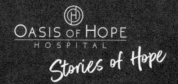

九地

TWELVE

TACKLE RESISTANCE

*For it is the soldier's disposition to offer
an obstinate resistance when surrounded.*

—Sun Tzu
The Art of War
The Nine Situations

—May 26, 1940. Dunkirk, France.

Defeat was inevitable. Nazi forces employed the *Lightning War* strategy mobilizing tanks and infantry so rapidly that hundreds of thousands of British soldiers were pushed back against the sea.[1] With no way out, death was certain. The troops needed a miracle, but there was no hope of walking on water to escape. They dug foxholes in the dunes. The British soldiers resisted the onslaught of the Nazi attackers at best they could. But, it was the valor of average citizens that led to a miraculous turn of events.[2] Great Britain's proverbial stiff upper lip was apparent when its army faced being vanquished. Winston Churchill defiantly declared, "We shall not flag nor fail. We shall go on to the end. We shall fight in France and on the seas and oceans; we shall fight with growing confidence and growing strength in the air..."[3]

Churchill's words launched *Operation Dynamo* on the impossible mission to rescue British soldiers. The hope, in the best-case scenario, was to evacuate 45,000 soldiers from Dunkirk harbor. The Royal Air Force was highly effective and holding back the attacks of the German Luftwaffe Air Force. Still, the British Navy did not have enough ships to evacuate the tens of thousands of soldiers. The British Admiralty called on all good citizens of the Crown, to take any seaworthy watercraft and set off for Dunkirk to bring the boys home. A fleet of seven hundred ferries, lifeboats, private yachts and fishing boats braved the threats of torpedoes in the water, while bullets and bombs rained down from the skies. The British citizens didn't evacuate 45,000 troops; they brought 300,000 troops to safety.[4] This unprecedented evacuation of troops became a turning point in World War II.

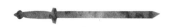

Thank God that Hitler had overlooked Sun Tzu's *Nine Situations of Battle*.[5] Had he studied the strategy, he would have known better than to keep pursuing the British Army once they reached Dunkirk. One of Sun Tzu's nine situations warned against backing an enemy into a corner with no exit. He observed that it was better not to drive an enemy into a place with no way out, because they would fight more ferociously once they realized they had lost all possibilities of escape. The more the aggressing army would advance against the enemy, the more resistant the enemy would become. British citizens' spirits became unbreakable in the face of German aggression. Because of Dunkirk, resolve to regroup and send their troops to war again ultimately led to victory with the help of the allied forces.

CANCER BECOMES RESISTANT

Something similar happens in the fight against cancer. The more a tumor is attacked, the more resistant it becomes. Tumors intrinsically resist attacks by cytotoxic drugs. But they also acquire resistance during treatment cycles. This combination of intrinsic resistance and acquired resistance makes beating cancer exceptionally challenging.

It's essential to vary tactics to undermine cancer's resistance. We explained how we change it up on cancer in chapter ten. Addressing a tumor's drug resistance is necessary to lower the risk of recurrence and spread. In this chapter, we will start with an overview of the various mechanisms tumors use to resist treatment. We will end with a review of therapies we employ to undermine cancer's resistance.

Cancer's intrinsic resistance, and acquired resistance, make it exceptionally difficult to defeat.

THE LAW OF DIMINISHING RETURNS

In economics, there is a law called *diminishing returns*. According to an article published in *The Economic Journal* in 1892, "The 'law' asserts that under certain circumstances, the returns to additional quantity of labour must necessarily diminish."[6] This law goes back to America's father of economics, Adam Smith and others. It explains how in agriculture, there is an optimum point of production. Beyond that, adding more labor and time starts to produce smaller and smaller outputs.

Some medical researchers have applied the law of diminishing returns to cancer treatment. The diminishing

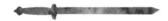

value of chemotherapy over repeated cycles is apparent in more than one way. First, patients are not able to tolerate the toxicity associated with the increased dosing.[7] Second, the more cancer is exposed to chemotherapy, the more resistant it becomes.

As we explained earlier, chemotherapy is very effective initially in many cancers. Unfortunately, most cancers will rebound and come back stronger. Then the drug that worked initially doesn't produce the same results in subsequent treatment. As outlined in chapter eight, a strength of cancer is that it can become resistant to treatments. It would take many books to explain the multiple molecular mechanisms involved in cytotoxic treatment resistance. Therefore, we will present a basic explanation.

A tumor's ability to develop treatment resistance is why chemotherapy ends up failing. It can also be a problem with natural therapies, but not nearly as pronounced as with conventional therapies. In a way, a tumor becoming resistant to treatment is like natural selection. The cancerous cells that have a mechanism that protects them from chemotherapy are the ones that survive and reproduce. A different mechanism is genetic—they mutate into drug-resistant cells. The increasing resistance of cancer is responsible for the diminishing returns when chemotherapy doses are increased.

HOW CANCER RESISTS TREATMENT

There are different ways malignant cells become resistant to treatment. The underlying threat comes from the cancerous cells that survive a particular chemotherapy. After treatment, only chemoresistant cells survive, and they reproduce more chemoresistant cells. But, even cells that don't have a drug-resistant nature can protect themselves.

CELL PUMPS

Healthy functioning cells exchange, share and pass forward ions, minerals and other molecules to each other.[8] Cells have specific proteins that function as pumps to do these tasks. Some cancer cells have proteins that work as a detox pump. In this way, the cell can protect itself from chemotherapy, and other cytotoxic agents by pumping them out. Several proteins boost cancer resistance. Major Vault Protein (MVP) has been found to help many types of cancer resist chemotherapy, including non-small cell lung carcinoma (NSCLC), B-cell lymphoma, glioma, leukemia and ovarian cancer. MXR1 is the protein that helps detox breast cancer cells of cytotoxic drugs.[9]

It is amazing that cells were designed with the capacity to detox themselves in this way. The human body truly is a marvel.

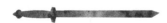

ONCOGENES

Oncogenes can help cancer cells become drug-resistant in direct and indirect ways. It's important to note that we are not only talking about "cancer genes" such as BRCA1. Normal genes can become oncogenic (cancer-promoting). Though it is not fully understood how genes can mutate and become oncogenic, a few molecular mechanisms are known. Apoptosis inhibition, cell signaling and encoding growth factor receptors are involved in gene mutation.[10] Comorbidities, such as obesity, contribute to genes mutating into oncogenes.

Here is the relationship between obesity and cancer. Adipokines are cytokines that are released from fatty connective tissue called adipose tissue. The upregulation of adipokines, such as adiponectin, leptin, and resistin, can result in MicroRNA becoming oncogenic.[11] MicroRNAs increase chemoresistance through transduction pathways in cancers of the lung, breasts, colon, prostate and ovaries.[12]

Epidermal growth factor receptor (EGFR) can also become an oncogene. EGFR is a protein-coding gene that is necessary for cells to proliferate and survive in normal physiology.[13] In many types of cancer, EGFR is over expressed.[14] EGFR can induce intratumoral angiogenic vasculature. The progeneration of new blood vessels is needed for tumors to thrive and progress. It also promotes intravasation of cells, which is instrumental in the spread of cancer and formation of metastases.[15]

EPITHELIAL-TO-MESENCHYMAL TRANSITION (EMT)

Epithelial-to-Mesenchymal Transition (EMT) increases cell survival in response to cytotoxic drugs because it downregulates Protease-Activated Response 4 (PAR-4). The PAR-4 gene normally encodes a tumor suppressor protein that targets cancer cells and induces apoptosis in the malignant cells. PAR-4 is often absent or mutated in cancers as a result of EMT. EMT increases drug resistance in multiple types of cancer including breast cancer and pancreatic cancer.[16]

DNA REPAIR

DNA has a tremendous capacity to repair itself. DNA repair helps cancerous cells survive after treatment with chemotherapy. Understand that chemotherapy can damage the DNA and RNA of mutated cells, which can halt their reproduction. As malignant cells repair their DNA after chemo-induced damage, they become increasingly resistant against chemotherapy. The two main pathways involved in DNA repair

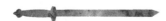

are nucleotide excision repair and mismatch repair. Both of these pathways recognize damage and then excise, resynthesize and replace the damaged DNA with the newly synthesized strand.[17]

AUTOPHAGY

Autophagy is a fundamental capacity of a cell to maintain its balance of energy. Autophagy can either increase the survival of a cell or induce its destruction (Autophagic programmed cell death). Autophagy increases cancer drug resistance by releasing exosomes and downregulating MicroRNAs.[18]

CANCER STEM CELLS

Stem cells have been in the news for the last ten years or so. They are the remarkable cells that can turn into any type of cell the body needs. A brain cell or a blood cell could develop out of the same stem cell. Imagine a stem that could bloom into whatever type of flower a garden needed. Unfortunately, there are cancer stem cells (CSC) too. They are primarily responsible for a recurrence of cancer after therapy has destroyed a tumor.

CSCs are in most tissues and avail themselves to all types of cancer, including breast, lung, ovarian, prostate, colon and leukemia. For chemotherapy and radiation to be effective, a tumor's microenvironment must have a sufficient oxygen level. Tumors are generally hypoxic. CSCs survive in deficient levels of oxygen. CSCs are so resistant to oxidative therapies that they are nearly untouchable. Another reason why CSCs are resistant to treatment is that chemotherapy acts on cells that are rapidly dividing by actively synthesizing DNA. CSCs are inactive and do not synthesize DNA. Thus, they are shielded from chemotherapy.[19] After a cycle of chemotherapy or radiation is completed, CSCs can regroup and form into new, more resistant, malignant cells that can form tumors and metastasize.

EXOSOMES

Exosomes, nano-sized vessels that mediate inter-cell communication, transfer proteins during tumorgenesis that can cause extrinsic therapy resistance. According to a recent study published in *Molecular Cancer,* exosomes are involved in many cancer resistance mechanisms. Exosomes transfer proteins that promote malignant cell DNA repair, generate CSCs through EMT, pump out intracellular drug concentrations and flush out proapoptotic proteins.[20] Exosomes can also transfer

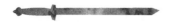

messages that can diminish immune surveillance of malignant cells by suppressing T cells, NK cells and dendritic cells.[21]

TACKLING RESISTANCE BY UNDERMINING IT

At the beginning of this chapter, we shared about one of the nine situations Sun Tzu writes about in *The Art of War*. The specific situation we are talking about is trapping an enemy and not leaving any route of escape. He warns of how the enemy will fight even harder when they realize their fate. Chemotherapy and radiation attack tumors directly and aggressively. They back cancer into a corner and try to kill it with the frontal attack.

At Oasis of Hope, our experience has shown us that direct attacks have diminishing returns, and aid and abet cancer becoming resistant. Instead, our approach is to undermine cancer. Our therapies and approach have the goal of excavating below the foundational strongholds of cancer. Instead of backing cancer into a corner, we dig out below it, causing it to lose its balance and topple over. One such stronghold is cancer's ability to become resistant to treatment. We leverage the metabolic traits of cancer and disarm its ability to regroup. Varying tactics has been effective in many cases. This method is what we call *the art and science of undermining cancer*.

Many of the therapies we employ at Oasis of Hope, serve in part to lower cancer's drug resistance. Let's conclude this chapter on undermining cancer resistance with three Ms and three Ns: Modulation, Metformin, metronomic dosing, nutrition, nanoceuticals and NF-κB inhibitors.

MODULATION

An essential strategy is to modulate therapies. We never give one type of treatment over and over again without changing it up. Instead, we modulate various types of treatments. We use our one-two-three-punch strategy that modulates to and from oxidative stress and antioxidative therapy. The main focus of modulating treatments is reactive oxygen species (ROS). ROS modulation is at the heart of our treatment. ROS are free radical molecules containing oxygen. Tumors typically have ROS levels that can be damaging and cause an imbalance between cellular reduction-oxidation (redox) conditions. Redox is favorable for cancer cell proliferation, angiogenesis, metastasis and a defective antioxidant system within cancerous cells that protects them.[22] Though it is generally accepted that free radicals, such as ROS, are associated with chronic diseases, increasing ROS levels can selectively kill cancer cells.

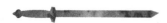

Oasis of Hope employs therapies, such as Ozone and HDIVC, to elevate ROS levels and break the redox homeostasis. Then, we change it up to modulate redox. Before tumors become resistant to our oxidative treatments, we hit them with specific antioxidants that help suppress NF-κB activation stimulated by cells with higher levels of ROS.[23]

METFORMIN

Metformin, developed initially to help control type II diabetes, has been widely studied for its ability to suppress oncogenesis and inhibit cancer stem cell activity. Cancer stem cells are associated with metastasis, drug resistance and cancer recurrence.[24] We will provide a comprehensive explanation of how Metformin works in chapter fifteen.

METRONOMIC DOSING

Studies demonstrate that tumors are more affected by the density of chemotherapy more than the quantity. Low-dose metronomic chemotherapy is a way to deliver less toxic doses at a higher frequency rate over an extended period. The cancer-killing effect is not initially apparent, due to the low dose (between 1/10 and 1/3 of maximum tolerable dose). But over time, it can be more effective at tumor destruction. Delivering small amounts frequently over time results in a higher density of treatment that is not as toxic as standard chemotherapy.

Another advantage of low-dose chemotherapy is that oral tablets are effective. Tablets are less expensive, have no treatment administration fee and can be taken at home. As far as the topic of resistance is concerned, the primary benefit of low-dose metronomic chemotherapy is that it can be given over an extended period.[25]

NUTRITION

You will read throughout our book that nutrition is the foundation of our cancer treatment. After successful treatment, nutrition and lifestyle are the only ways to maintain long-term cancer-free living. You will need to make a full commitment to keeping on a healthy diet, exercising and managing stress.

Nutrients from a whole food plant-based diet can help against cancer drug resistance. Studies show that a diet rich in polyphenols has anticancer qualities.[26] Our plant-based diet includes polyphenol-rich foods, such as vegetables, fruits, whole grains, nuts, olive oil and tea. Polyphenols combat cancer drug resistance by detoxing carcinogens, promoting apoptosis and modulating ROS. We recommend foods rich in the specific polyphenols EGCG, genistein, lycopene, curcumin, quercetin

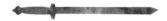

and resveratrol. Each of these polyphenols has different anticancer effects, including anti-inflammation, miRNA modulation, upregulation of the tumor suppressor genes p53 and Rb, and the suppression of cancer stem cells self-renewal activity.[27]

Polyphenols, such as sulforaphane, are potent CSC activity suppressors. Sulforaphane is found in higher concentrations in cruciferous vegetables such as broccoli, kale, cabbage and bok choy.[28] It is also important to note that the Oasis of Hope diet is based on low glycemic index foods. Avoiding foods with a high GI helps disrupt the CSC metabolism, which is predominantly glycolytic; though CSCs can also gain energy via oxidative phosphorylation.[29]

The Oasis of Hope plant-based polyphenol-rich diet supports healthy cell metabolism and disrupts a malignant cell metabolism. Nutrients from whole foods are the most bioavailable to our bodies. For prevention, we promote nutrition over supplements. For cancer treatment, studies confirm that not all nutrients can be absorbed in the levels needed for the full anticancer effect. We have proprietary nanoceuticals to provide therapeutic doses that can be absorbed by the cells.

NANOCEUTICALS

There are more than five thousand nutrients that can turn oncogenes on or off. There are several challenges to overcome to use nutrients to undermine cancer effectively. They include identifying the right nutrients, determining effective dosing and facilitating absorption. As for the first challenge, we have a team of researchers led by our applied nutritionist, Mark McCarty. He, and the other researchers, scour through the latest findings published in peer-reviewed medical journals. Their work keeps us on the leading edge of cancer-fighting nutrients and treatments.

When it comes to the challenges of dosing and absorption, it is often difficult for a person to consume enough nutrients presented in capsules to achieve an effective dose. It is common for patients to take between thirty and sixty capsules of nutraceuticals each day. The way we overcome this challenge is through nanotechnology.

Nanoceuticals are nutrients that have been transformed into nanoparticles. A nanometer is one-billionth of a meter. Our nutrients are less than one hundred nanometers in size. A sheet of paper is one hundred thousand nanometers thick. Our nutrients are one thousand times smaller than the thickness of a sheet of paper, or a strand of human hair.

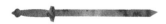

We have carefully formulated nanoceuticals in the form of liposomal emulsions. How does this help with absorption? Clinical evidence shows that nanoformulations improve bioavailability, protect against the degradation of nutrients and diminish negative side effects such as nausea.[30] They provide nutrients in therapeutic doses with better absorption. Instead of taking sixty capsules, we can deliver the anticancer nutrients in less than a tablespoon of liquid mixed into juice or water. Let's take a look at a number of the nanonutrients we provide that are specific to lowering cancer resistance:

- **Curcumin** lowers cancer resistance to capecitabine (Xeloda), a prodrug that is converted to 5FU in the liver and malignant cells. Curcumin is also highly effective at destroying cancer stem cells, which are essential for disease recurrence.[31]
- **Silybum Marianum** inhibits multidrug resistance-associated proteins. It also potentiates chemo drugs and protects the liver from chemo.[32]
- **Green Tea** lowers the risk of cancers of the stomach, esophagus and lung. It also lowers drug resistance because it is highly concentrated in the polyphenol EGCG. EGCG causes strong chemopreventive effects by regulating or inhibiting occurs through its regulation of VEGF, EGFR, MMPs and NF-κB.[33]
- **Grape Seed Extract**'s proanthocyanidin polyphenol lowers drug resistance, induces apoptosis and suppresses carcinogenic activities by modulating miRNA and cytokine expression.[34]
- **Resveratrol** is the best-known polyphenol that promotes heart health. Resveratrol is anti-carcinogenic and lowers cancer resistance through the modulation of glycolysis.[35]
- **Boswella Serrata** has the therapeutic actions of anti-inflammation, inducing apoptosis and suppressing DNA synthesis in cancer cells.[36]
- **Selenium**'s primary chemopreventive quality is that it induces apoptosis in malignant cells.[37] It has additional anticancer qualities including redox regulation, immune modulation and cell detoxification.[38]

- **Zinc** suppresses DNA repair in malignant cells, which inhibits cancer development caused by DNA damage.[39]
- **Glycine**'s mechanism of lowering resistance is not precisely known. Still, studies indicate it helps maintain redox homeostasis, which is associated with treatment sensitivity.[40]
- **Omega 3** is vital in cancer treatment. It is a potent anti-inflammatory, an excellent adjuvant to oxidative therapies, and it lowers drug resistance by suppressing proinflammatory gene expression.[41]
- **CoenzymeQ10** does not exhibit chemopreventive qualities, but it does protect healthy cells from damage caused by chemotherapy and radiation, and it is shown to help with treatment fatigue.[42]
- **Vitamin D₃** is chemopreventive because it lowers autophagy and suppresses NF-κB.[43]

NF-κB INHIBITORS

The suppression of NF-κB is such an important factor in cancer treatment. We dedicated a significant portion of chapter seven to the strategy. We won't repeat what we already presented. Still, we will mention a couple of additional important points about lowering cancer's drug resistance by inhibiting NF-κB. One of cancer's metabolic traits is that its microenvironment is hypoxic. Hypoxia-inducible factor-1 (HIF-1) promotes EMT, which increases cancer's proliferation, angiogenesis and chemoresistance. The upregulation of NF-κB is also associated with cytotoxic drug resistance. Studies support our three for one strategy of using salicylates to inhibit NF-κB, which suppresses HIF-1, which in turn downregulates EMTs. Salicylates help lower drug resistance and promote apoptosis in malignant cells.

Celebrex and Alin are quite effective at inhibiting NF-κB activation.[44] We inhibit NF-κB activation further with our nanoceuticals containing curcumin, EGCG, silibinin and resveratrol.[44-48]

CONCLUSION

In this chapter, we shared that the more cancer is attacked, the more resilient it becomes. We outlined numerous mechanisms that cancer has to become resistant to treatment. We also explained six of the main strategies we use to lower a tumor's resistance to treatment. In the next chapter, we will discuss the different stages of cancer and how we make adjustments to our treatment protocols based on the stage of cancer and the condition of the patient.

STORY OF HOPE

Merry Trujillo • Breast Cancer • 2001

My name is Merry Trujillo. In June of 2001, my primary care physician referred me to University Medical Center, Las Vegas, because a malignant mass was found in my left breast. The tests gave me the diagnosis as follows:

> Invasive ductal carcinoma, associated with extensive intraductal carcinoma of comedo carcinoma and cribriform types. Tumor size 2.0 x 1.5 x 1.3 cm. All margins negative. Extensive calcifications within the intraductal component. Vascular invasion identified.

I was given just six months to live. I decided to go to Oasis of Hope Hospital because my son-in-law in Nicaragua had a family member that had received treatment there. From the first moment I arrived at the hospital, I felt I could trust the doctors. I received professional care at all times.

In my first year of treatment, I never had radiation or chemotherapy. After fifteen months, I went into remission. I would return to Oasis of Hope every three months for a follow-up exam. Nineteen years later, I continue to be cancer-free thanks to God.

—Mery Trujillo
Henderson, Nevada
USA

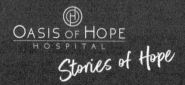

地形

THIRTEEN

TREAT BY STAGE

If you know the enemy and know yourself,
your victory will not stand in doubt;
if you know Heaven and know Earth,
you may make your victory complete.

—Sun Tzu
The Art of War
Terrain

King Leonidas led three hundred Spartan warriors against King Xerxes' tens of thousands of soldiers in the *Battle of Thermopylae*. How did the Spartans hold the Persians back for three days against impossible odds? They used the terrain. Thermopylae was a narrow passageway, a chokepoint, where only a few hundred troops could pass through together. Xerxes sent wave after wave of soldiers against the Spartans, but because of the chokepoint, Leonidas and his men only had to fight a few hundred enemy troops at any given moment. This battle took place four hundred and eight years before Christ.[1] Chances are, you became aware of this battle when *Legendary Films* and *Warner Brothers* released the film *300* back in 2007.[2] The graphically violent movie clearly demonstrated how terrain is a determining factor in war. The same is true in the battle against cancer.

General Sun Tzu had a strategy for narrow passes, just like King Leonidas used to his advantage at Thermopylae. Sun Tzu stated, "With regard to narrow passes, if you can occupy them first, let them be strongly garrisoned and await the advent of the enemy."[3] Leonidas leveraged this strategy, and it proved to work in Sparta as it had worked for Sun Tzu in China. Effective war strategies proved on the battlefield can be adapted and adopted for other types of challenges like business and healthcare.

How could the concept of adjusting the fight to the topographical conditions of different terrains be applied in oncology? Imagine that in the fight against cancer, we look at its different stages and aggressiveness as variations in terrain. The plan of attack must be changed depending on the stage and variables.

Sun Tzu recognized that war tactics needed to be adapted to the type of terrain his army would face. He wrote that some

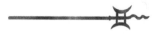

land is very accessible and can be freely traversed. Stage one cancer is like that type of land. It is accessible and quite easy to treat with a high cure rate. Some ground can be hard to take back if lost. In cancer, metastasis would be a terrain that is hard to take back.

Some land is better left alone because it presents no advantage to either side. Terrain that is better left alone could be slow-progressing cancers that pose no real threat. For example, we don't treat low-grade (Gleason 3+3) prostate cancer aggressively because the cure rate is high and very rarely progresses to the point that it takes the patient's life.

Let's set the groundwork for this chapter. We will discuss early detection, screening methods, the difference between operable and inoperable cancers, and cancer staging. We will wrap the chapter up explaining how we vary our treatment protocols depending on the stage and aggressiveness of different cancer types.

EARLY DETECTION & EARLY DIAGNOSIS ARE KEY

The survivability of cancer has increased. Over the last twenty years, survival rates have increased in eleven of the sixteen most common cancer types in men and thirteen of the eighteen most common cancer types in women.[4] Though this is great news, the gains have been made in early-stage cancers.

Improvement in cancer survivability is mostly due to early detection and early diagnosis, not improvements in treatment. Studies find that early diagnosis is the primary factor for survival. As published in the *British Journal of Cancer*, "Optimal and 'curative' treatment can only be offered to patients diagnosed at an early enough stage to benefit from it."[5]

Early detection and early diagnosis are not always possible. Cancer is often a silent disease, and many people are diagnosed when the cancer is already in an advanced stage.

Let's take a moment to talk about screening. If you are reading this and have cancer, you will want this information for your loved ones! Screening is not preventative. Screening is for detection. In other words, screening will either tell you that no cancer is detected, or it will detect cancer, hopefully in an early stage. A mammogram will never prevent breast cancer, and it can increase cancer risk slightly as it uses radiation to make the image. The risk can be reduced almost to zero by having one every other year, instead of annually.[6]

For your family members who don't have cancer, screening is important, because if cancer is detected and diagnosed in an early stage, the probability of cure is high. Screening becomes

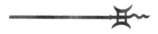

increasingly important as we age because the incidence of cancer increases as we grow older.

When it comes to preventing cancer, lifestyle changes are your best bet. Healthy nutrition, exercise and stress management are effective preventive measures.

Breast self-examination is an important early detection tool.

BREAST SELF-EXAMINATION, ULTRASOUND & MAMMOGRAPHY

For breast cancer detection, breast self-examination is an effective method that is completely radiation free.[7] Though breast self-examination is not correlated to increased survival rates, it is effective for discovering a lump, which leads to seeking a medical evaluation earlier.[8]

Ultrasound is another radiation-free screening tool for breast cancer. According According to the *Journal of Global Oncology*, ultrasound effectively detects palpable abnormalities and distinguishes between cysts and solid masses.[9] We recommend that women below the age of fifty use breast self-examination and ultrasound (also called a sonogram) instead of mammography to reduce radiation exposure. Another advantage of ultrasound is that it works better in dense breast tissue than mammography.[10] This option is especially suitable for younger women as they tend to have dense breast tissue. We recommend screening for breast cancer by self-examination and ultrasounds starting at age twenty. To avoid exposing breasts to radiation, we only recommend mammograms when an ultrasound detects something suspicious. For women over the age of fifty, a mammogram every other year is sufficient.

MRI

An excellent diagnostic machine for detecting tumors, whether benign or malignant, is the whole-body magnetic resonance imaging (MRI). This technology uses a high power magnet to create the image instead of radiation. It has demonstrated to be as effective at a CT scan in many tumors, except for cancers of the pituitary gland, colon and lung.[11] The main drawback of using an MRI annually is the cost.

We don't recommend MRI for breast cancer screening because it often results in false positives, and many centers do not have the specialized magnets or antennas required for a breast study. Advancements in MRI technology could make it the choice for cancer screening of breast cancer in the future.

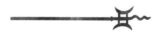

DIGITAL RECTAL EXAM

We recommend an annual check-up, including a digital rectal exam (DRE) for men over the age of forty. A DRE works well for detecting abnormalities in the prostate and rectum.[12] If a primary physician detects something out of the norm, a patient should be referred to a urologists for additional testing.

COLONOSCOPY

A colonoscopy is the best method for screening for colorectal cancer. An inspection of the colon is conducted by inserting an endoscopic camera through the rectum into the colon. If any precancerous polyps are found, they can be removed as a part of the examination and sent to pathology for further evaluation.[13] Polyps should be removed as a preventive measure because they often become malignant. You should have your first colonoscopy by age forty-five. It is recommended to have a colonoscopy once every ten years between the ages of forty-five and seventy-five.[14] The benefits must be weighed against the risks for colonoscopy for people over the age of seventy-five. Complications resulting from the procedure are more common in elderly individuals.[15]

CHEST X-RAY & CT SCAN

A simple chest x-ray is inexpensive and can detect abnormalities in the lungs.[16] An x-ray is not sufficient to diagnose lung cancer, but it can be an excellent screening method to determine if further studies should be conducted. A Computed Tomography (CT) scan is more effective for detecting lung cancer. Though quite effective at identifying tumors where cancer is present, we do not recommend CT scans for screening purposes due to the expense and radiation exposure risks. A CT scan is advisable for people presenting symptoms of lung cancer syndrome, and for high-risk patients such as heavy smokers experiencing symptoms of lung disease.[17]

FDG-PET/CT SCAN

The most useful imaging tool available for cancer detection and evaluation is a Positron Emission Tomography, with glucose analog 2-Fluoro-2-Deoxy-d-Glucose, combined with Computed Tomography (FDG-PET/CT). It is very precise in identifying the anatomic location of tumors.[18] The CT scan creates the image of the organs throughout the body. FDG is the sugary radioactive substance that the PET scan lights up.

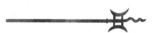

Tumor's have and affinity for glucose, so the FDG gets highly concentrated within malignant cells. PET scans create images of biochemical and physiologic activity. This technology is often capable of distinguishing between benign and malignant tissues that CT scans alone cannot.[19] Two drawbacks of a PET/CT scan are the exposure to radiation and the high expense. Some people will opt for using at PET/CT scan as a screening tool for early detection because studies conclude that it is fourteen times more effective at detecting malignancies than any other imaging technology.[20] We don't promote the use of such an expensive technology for screening. Instead, we use this vital technology for diagnostic purposes and to monitor disease progression.

TUMOR MARKERS

Screening technology cannot detect all types of cancer. In the case of ovarian cancer, no screening test has proved effective for early detection, though it will show up on PET scans.[21] In cancers that don't show up with imaging technology, we turn to blood tests known as tumor markers. Tumor markers are defined as "Measurable biochemicals that are associated with a malignancy. These markers are either produced by tumor cells (tumor-derived) or by the body in response to tumor cell growth (tumor-associated)."[22] Most tumor markers detect the presence of cancer-associated antigens or hormones. But these biochemicals can also be related to illnesses other than cancer. For this reason, tumor markers are generally not used for definitive diagnosis of cancer. Take the prostate-specific antigen (PSA). An elevated level doesn't mean that a person has cancer of the prostate. An higher than normal PSA can also signal an infection of the prostate, urinary tract infection, or the extremely common benign prostatic hyperplasia (BPH). This is why there is a significant problem with over-diagnosing people with prostate cancer based on higher than normal PSA values.[23]

Tumor markers are best suited for monitoring cancer progression based on changes in their levels over time. Below, you will find the types of tumor markers we commonly use.

Tumor Marker	Abbreviation	Cancer Type
Cancer antigen 125	CA125	Ovarian
Cancer antigen 15-3	CA15-3	Breast
Cancer antigen 19-9	CA19-9	Pancreatic
Carcinoembryonic antigen	CEA	Colorectal, pancreatic, breast & gastric
Prostate-specific antigen	PSA	Prostate
Human Chorionic Gonadotropin	HCG	Testicular
Alpha-fetoprotein	AFP	Liver

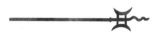

BIOPSY

Biopsies are never used as a screening tool because they are invasive. Some studies indicate that they may have some risk of releasing cancer cells into the bloodstream, which could lead to metastases.[24] When imaging studies show a tumor or suspicious mass, a biopsy is the only definitive diagnostic tool to confirm a malignancy and cancer type.[25] The two most common methods of biopsy are surgical removal of tissue or fine needle aspiration (FNA) of tissue. The surgeon will choose the method depending on the location and accessibility of the tumor.

OPERABLE CANCER VS. INOPERABLE CANCER

When a patient is first diagnosed with cancer, the first instinct is to want a surgical oncologist to cut it out. In a case that removing a tumor would result in a cure, it would be the logical, moral and ethical thing to do. If the tumor is inoperable, surgery is not a viable option. So what determines if a tumor is operable or inoperable?

Good surgical practice starts with an assessment of the size, location and anatomic involvement of the tumor. The first thing to determine is if the patient will survive the surgery. The next step is to determine how the surgery will affect the patient's quality of life. The benefits and risks a surgery presents to the patient are weighed to evaluate the operability, or resectability of a tumor.[26]

In chapter ten, we went into depth about preserving the quality of life of a patient, and avoiding aggressive surgeries like the commando and hemicorporectomy. So here, we just want to provide some definitions of operable and inoperable cancer.

Cancer is considered operable when the surgery presents a high probability of cure. For example, localized renal cancer is considered operable. Renal cancer is localized if the tumor is encapsulated in the kidney and has not spread to surrounding tissue or distant organs. The recommended procedure is a radical nephrectomy that involves removing the affected kidney, the attached adrenal gland, nearby lymph nodes, and the fatty tissue around the kidney. The five-year survival rate after surgery for localized cancer of the kidney is ninety-three percent.[27] Considering the quality of life, a patient can live a completely healthy life with one kidney. The risks are minimal, and the probability of cure is high, which is a perfect example of operable cancer.

There are two reasons why a tumor would be considered inoperable. The first one is obvious. If a tumor cannot be removed without killing the patient, then it is inoperable. An

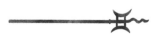

example of this would be brainstem gliomas.[28] It is impossible to perform the surgery successfully. The patient will not survive.

The other reason why cancer would be categorized as inoperable is less apparent. There are many cases where surgery can be done, and the patient would survive, but the tumor is still inoperable. Why? In cancer surgery, "inoperable" doesn't only mean that it can't be done, like in brainstem gliomas. It can also mean that the surgery does not present a high probability of cure.

An example of this would be stage IV breast cancer in which cancer has metastasized to the bone or another organ. Removing the primary tumor in the breast does not increase the probability of survival. A tumor is inoperable if doing the surgery does not increase the probability of cure, even if the surgery could be done. In advanced-stage breast cancer, oncologists recommend combination therapy of chemotherapy and radiation, known as chemoradiation, and hormone therapy instead of surgery.[29] Oasis of Hope has many non-toxic alternatives to off patients with stage IV cancer of the breast. Our protocols have led to the highest five-year survival rates for stage IV breast cancer anywhere.

OPERATING ON THE INOPERABLE

There are often cases in which surgery will be programmed even if the tumor is inoperable. The two main reasons such a procedure would be done would be to save the patient from an imminent life-threatening condition, or to improve the patient's quality of life. For example, if cancer is causing a bowel obstruction that could provoke ischemia or a perforation, emergency surgery must be done, or the patient will likely die.[30] Resecting the colon won't increase the probability of cancer cure—therefore, the cancer is inoperable—but the surgery is necessary to save the patient's life. Some surgeries are required to help a patient live to fight another day. In this same example, the surgery will significantly improve the patient's quality of life by alleviating the excruciating pain associated with bowel obstruction. This type of surgery is referred to as palliative because it alleviates pain and improves the quality of life without treating the disease. Debulking is an example of a palliative surgery.

Debulking of an inoperable tumor may present advantages to a patient. For example, in the case of ovarian cancer, debulking may not improve the probability of cure. Still, studies indicate that it does increase the disease-free interval in most patients before a recurrence is experienced.[31] Increasing the

disease-free interval is vital because ovarian cancer has a recurrence rate of seventy percent. If a debulking surgery can be done, increasing the time a person can live before recurrence is very beneficial. At Oasis of Hope, we can take advantage of the extra time do provide a number of our therapies that could help control cancer. Debulking can improve the prognosis by buying time for other therapies to work, alleviating pain and relieving emotional distress. Let me tell you about Bob.

BOB THE TUMOR

We had a patient with advanced carcinoma of the ovary. She had come to the clinic after being treated with chemotherapy for an extended period. After four lines of chemotherapy failed, she was sent home to die because there was nothing else that could be done. Her tumor was so big that people mistakenly thought she was pregnant and asked when she was due. When she came to Oasis of Hope, her condition was very poor, as was her prognosis. We started her on our *Core* therapy. It was quite effective, and the tumor reduced in size by nearly fifty percent. The reduction was enough that a debulking surgery could be considered.

The patient was so excited, and she told me, "Well, I think it's now time for Bob to be born." I asked her, "Bob? What are you talking about?" "Well, people have asked me so often if I'm pregnant, that I decided to call the tumor 'Bob.'" After four months of *Core* therapy and home therapy, debulking was possible. We took her into surgery and removed the enormous tumor. Baby Bob weighed eleven pounds and was born by cesarean. (Remember: It was a tumor, not a baby. It was debulking, not a C-section!)

The debulking surgery removed nearly one hundred percent of the tumor. She responded well, the tumor markers went down, and the tumor never came back. Though the surgery was not curative, it brought great relief to our patient. By taking out the eleven-pound mass, her quality of life improved dramatically. She was able to walk better, breathe normally, and experience an incredible reduction in pain and discomfort. There was another critical outcome. Her body no longer had to fight the massive tumor and began to respond even better to our *Core* therapy. Soon she was completely healed. She lived many years after and died of old age, not cancer.

This is a prime example of when integrative therapy, or complementary therapy, is the best for a patient. The combination of our therapy with surgery was very effective. It resulted in giving her many extra years of quality living.

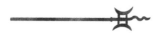

NEOADJUVANT THERAPY

Another strategy we use with inoperable tumors is neoadjuvant therapy. The primary objective of neoadjuvant therapy is to reduce the size of an inoperable tumor enough that it becomes operable. Consider a patient with breast cancer who is scheduled for a mastectomy. Neoadjuvant therapy could make a patient a lumpectomy candidate, which would avoid the loss of the breast and the need for breast reconstruction.[32] The therapy is not curative, but it reduces the size of the tumor, saves the patient's breast and dramatically improves the quality of life.

The most common neoadjuvant therapies are combinations of chemotherapies and radiation. Oasis of Hope combination therapies of HDIVC, Ozone, Hyperthermia, amygdalin and DCV often achieve the same benefits of neoadjuvant therapies without adverse side effects. Alternatives to chemotherapy and radiation are needed as conventional neoadjuvant therapies offer few benefits for some types of cancer. For example, though surgery will not be curative in pancreatic cancer, it will increase the length of survival much better than neoadjuvant therapy.[33]

Oasis of Hope neoadjuvant therapies can make advanced-stage cancers more treatable.

We are approaching the midpoint of this chapter, so let's pick up the theme of adapting to the terrain again. At the beginning of the chapter, we talked about how the different stages of cancer are like different terrains. Some terrain is easy for the army to fight on. Some terrain is better left alone. Some terrain, if lost, is hard to get back. So let's take a close look at the staging of cancer and how Oasis of Hope adapts our treatment protocols depending on the stage and aggressiveness of a cancer.

STAGING

Staging cancer is necessary because it will help determine how best to vary protocols depending on what stage the cancer is and how aggressive it is. One thing that we would like to emphasize here is that late-stage cancers have many possibilities to be treated with favorable outcomes. Interventions need to be adapted according to stage.

To help understand how we stage cancers, here is a table, based on a chart developed by the National Cancer Institute.[34] We added more information to clearly explain how most tumors are staged.

Stages of Cancer

Stage	Explanation
Stage 0	Malignant cells are present, but they have not spread to surrounding tissue.
Stage I	The primary tumor is less than 2 cm large. Cancer has not spread to distant parts of the body.
Stage II	The primary tumor is ≥ 2cm large, or malignant cells have spread to surrounding tissue and/or lymph nodes.
Stage III	The primary tumor is more than 5 cm, or it is 2.5 cm to 4.5 cm and has spread to the surrounding lymph nodes.
Stage IV	Cancer has spread to distant parts of the body to form tumors other than the primary tumor. A distant tumor is called a "metastasis."

Referencing the definitions from the table on the previous page, we will take several types of cancer and describe how we treat each of them, depending on the stage and other variables. Again, just as General Sun Tzu used various tactics depending on the terrain, we will share how we vary tactics deepening on the stage and aggressiveness of a tumor. Let's start with early stage cancers and move on from there.

EARLY STAGE CANCERS

Some cancers have high cure rates with conventional therapies when they are in an early stage. In those cases, alternatives are not necessary. For a tumor is stage one, surgery is the best course of action. A tumor that can be removed completely has a very high rate of cure. For stage one cancers of the breast, lung, kidney and stomach, we recommend surgery.

Pancreatic cancer is the only stage one cancer that we hesitate to recommend surgery. The *Whipple Procedure* is a massive surgery in which close to seventy-five percent of the stomach is removed. The duodenum and gallbladder are removed, along with part of the gall ducts and the bile ducts. Then a reconstruction of what is left after the aggressive removal of organs is done. The morbidity and mortality for this surgery are extremely high. About one in four will die of sepsis. One studied stated, "The magnitude of the surgical stress of this procedure and the (compromised) functional reserve of this patient population can be a notable factor influencing the outcome."[35] Though we have excellent techniques and anesthesia, it is such an aggressive surgery that we don't often recommend it. Even when a patient survives the procedure, the quality of life is compromised after so many organs are removed. With pancreatic cancer, we get better results with our therapy than surgery, even in early stages.

There are some other early stage cancers that surgery is not the best first option. In the case of tumors in the lower rectum or the anus, we try therapies other than surgery. The standard procedure in those cases is the removal of the rectum and

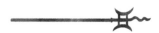

placement of colostomy. For rectal and anal cancer, just as with pancreatic cancer, we opt for alternatives to surgery. Quality of life considerations guide us. In most types of cancer, whenever we can remove a tumor, surgery is the option.

After surgeries are done, preventive therapies are administered because cancer recurs in twenty to thirty percent of stage one cancers. Conventional oncologists usually recommend adjuvant chemotherapy or radiation following surgery. Though often effective, conventional treatments have adverse side effects and harm the immune system.

Following surgery with Oasis of Hope *Core* or *Enhanced* therapies could be as effective as chemotherapy or radiotherapy, without the negative side effects. Oasis of Hope protocols are designed to preserve the quality of life, boost the immune system and protect against a cancer recurrence.

With cancers in stages two and three, we try to convert them to stage one and then surgically remove because the cure rate is high for operable stage one cancer. For example, in stage one cancer of the colon, the cure rate is eighty percent. In stage two is about sixty-eight percent. In stage three, it is about forty-five percent.[36] If cancer can be brought back to stage one before operating, it's advantageous to the patient. As explained before, neoadjuvant therapies of chemotherapy, radiation, or the combination called chemoradiation therapy, are generally employed to try to convert stage two and three cancers back to stage one.

Oasis of Hope's neoadjuvant therapies are natural and non-toxic. We are often successful in bringing cancer back to an earlier stage with our *Core* therapy. Our *Enhanced* therapy could be even more effective because it includes our dendritic cell vaccine. If a tumor becomes operable, we do a surgery followed by more treatment to reduce recurrence significantly. Our combination therapy may include neoadjuvant therapy, surgery and adjuvant therapy, which provide tremendous advantages over chemoradiation therapy.

ADVANCED-STAGE CANCERS

The National Cancer Institute (NCI) defines advanced cancer as "Cancer that is unlikely to be cured or controlled with treatment. Cancer may have spread from where it first started to nearby tissue, lymph nodes, or distant parts of the body. Treatment may be given to help shrink the tumor, slow the growth of cancer cells, or relieve symptoms."[37] Advanced-stage cancers are also called *metastatic cancer*. Once cancer has metastasized, it is generally considered to be in stage IV.

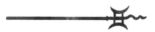

A metastasis occurs when cancerous cells, from the primary tumor, travel to another organ in the body and form a tumor.[38] The malignant cells in a metastasis are the same as the primary tumor. In other words, if a person has adenocarcinoma of the breast, and it spreads to the liver and forms a tumor there, the new tumor in the liver is a breast cancer tumor, not a liver cancer tumor.

HOPE TO UNDERMINE & OVERCOME STAGE IV CANCER

Once cancer has metastasized, it is very tough to treat. That's why the NCI states that advanced cancer has a very low probability of cure or control. We present this information simply to explain why Oasis of Hope has become a center known for helping patients facing stage IV cancer though it is challenging.

The American Cancer Society projected survival statistics for 2020 inspire hope. It states that the five-year survival rate for all cancer types and stages combined is eighty-five percent. This great news is due to early detection and early diagnosis. Two things happen when cancer is caught early. First, as we explained above, cancers in early stages are often operable, which means that if the tumor is completely removed, the probability of cure is eighty percent or more.

The second impact early detection has on survival statistics is giving a longer lead-time on tracking the patient's survival time.[39] Survival times can be confusing because two patients could have the same cancer that started on the same date. If they both lived seven years after being diagnosed, they could still have two different survival times on record. Imagine that the first patient had a screening and found cancer within the first year of the tumor forming, and he lived another six years. He would be grouped into the five-year survival category. If the second patient discovered the tumor in its fifth year since it first started forming, and lived two years from the time of diagnosis, he would be put in the two-year survival category. Both patients had the same timeline and type of cancer, but the earlier detected cancer showed a longer survival rate. Let's just put it this way. Statistics are confusing and up to interpretation. So let us encourage you by making this uplifting statement:

You are not a statistic!

We will never look at you as a statistic. We use statistics to help us provide optimal treatment options. We cannot go by statistics alone because cancer evolves differently in each

person. If the overall five-year survival for all types of cancer is eighty-five percent, why does cancer seem insurmountable? It's precisely because stage IV cancers have alarmingly low survival rates. Consider the differences between stage I and stage IV five-year survival rates for some of the more common cancer types published by the NCI.[40]

Cancer Type	Stage I 5-Year Survival Rate	Stage IV Five-Year Survival Rate
Breast	99%	27%
Ovary	92%	29%
Lung	19%	5%
Colorectal	90%	13%

These statistics demonstrate that early detection is responsible for prolonged survival. Look how significant the drop off is for stage IV cancers. The next chart compares the five-year survival rates in stage IV cancers when treated with conventional therapy versus being treated with Oasis of Hope *Core* therapy. These results were published in the medical publication *The Townsend Letter*.[41]

Cancer Type	Five-Year Survival Rate Conventional	Five-Year Survival Rate Oasis of Hope
Breast	27%	45%
Ovary	29%	54%
Lung	5%	9%
Colon	13%	16%

More than eighty-five percent of our patients at Oasis of Hope have stage IV cancer. They have already suffered severe negative side effects, have been significantly debilitated and had their immune systems devastated by chemotherapy or radiation. Conventional treatment centers start with patients that have not been harmed by any previous therapy. Still, their five-year survival rates are significantly lower than ours.

Critics of Oasis of Hope will often say that we give false hope and promise cures to incurable cancer. If you are this far into the book, you can witness that we never promise a cure. The hope we offer is one demonstrated by published results from our prospective study. If you have stage IV cancer and see that the probability of five-year survival with chemo and radiation is twenty-seven percent, but at Oasis of Hope it is forty-five percent, doesn't that inspire hope? What about the quality of life? Even if our five-year survival rate were the same as conventional treatments, but we could get the results without causing the severe adverse side effects associated with chemo and radiation, wouldn't that inspire hope?

Would it be false hope to share the five-year survival rate for stage IV ovary cancer is twenty-nine percent with conventional treatment and fifty-four percent with Oasis of Hope treatments? Again, we clearly are not promising anyone a cure.

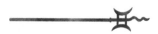

We are stating that fifty-four percent of stage IV ovarian cancer patients are expected to live at least five years.

Does the statistic that only nine percent of our stage IV lung cancer patients live at least five years look hopeless? That number is low, but considering that the national average survival rate for stage IV lung cancer is only five percent, many people prefer to give Oasis of Hope a try. No matter how long we can extend a patient's life, we work tirelessly to improve their quality of life. Helping people extend life, and live the days they have to the fullest, is the most hope-inspiring thing about the Oasis of Hope treatment experience.

When it comes to stage IV colon cancer, the improvement in the quality of life is the most important reason to choose Oasis of Hope for treatment. Even though our five-year survival rate is only three percent higher than the national average published by the NCI, the quality of life we can provide our patients is priceless.

HOW WE ACHIEVE BETTER RESULTS

There is not a short answer to explain how we have been able to achieve better results. It would take writing a book and providing hundreds of references from peer-reviewed medical journals to share how we get superior results. Oh, wait. We already wrote the book, and you are reading it now, LOL. Let us take a moment to highlight the key strategies we implement in our Oasis of Hope *Core* and Oasis of Hope *Enhanced* treatments. These strategies make up the art and science of undermining cancer. This book explains our strategies to undermine cancer including evaluation, planning, use of synergistic therapies, defending against the strengths of cancer, hitting cancer where it is vulnerable, using some strong therapies to engage with force, changing things up to keep cancer off balance, mobilizing the immune system, tackling chemoresistance, treating cancer by stage, using the elements of earth, air, water and fire, and being vigilant to to increase longevity and prevent cancer recurrence. Oasis of Hope treatment plan elements

Our treatment plan provides a patient with these elements:

1. Evaluation & Assessment
2. Treatment Planning
3. Detoxification
4. Preconditioning
5. Oxidative Therapies
6. Nutrition Therapy & Training
7. Emotional Support
8. Spiritual Healing
9. Immunotherapies
10. Lifestyle Education
11. Home Therapy with Anti-oxidants and Prodrugs
12. Follow-up Treatments

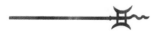

CONCLUSION

We hope the information on how we treat cancer by stages has been helpful. The wellness of our patients motivates our treatment recommendations. We want patients to achieve a life extension, but our primary focus is on helping our patients feel as well and strong as possible each day that is added to their lives.

We would like to end this chapter with the following testimony of on of our dear patients that has been in a long time fight. She came to us after multiple recurrences and we have had to make adjustments to our treatment objectives to improve the quality of life she has enjoyed. At this moment, we can't predict how long her life will be extended, but we know that her quality of life has been dramatically improved. Not all cancer testimonies are about a miraculous cure. Some are about the beautiful things that happen amid the struggle.

Not everyone will become as self-aware as our dear patient whose testimony we are sharing here. But, in the face of this massive challenge you are facing, you have the opportunity to grow in ways you have never imagined. We hope this story will inspire you to fight onward. It is anonymous as the struggle continues at the writing of this book.

MY CANCER JOURNEY

I first discovered I had ovarian cancer in 2013. I had a recurrence in 2015. I had another recurrence in 2018. That is what brought me to Oasis of Hope. I wasn't very surprised when cancer returned in 2018. I had a very stressful occurrence in my life that I could not get a handle on. No matter what I tried, I was filled with anger and resentment. I couldn't shake it. I was distressed and distraught for months and months. I didn't know what to do. I was also very aware that I was opening the door for illness and disease to return. When it came back, I was not surprised.

The first time that I had cancer, of course, I was very shocked. The doctor called me while I was driving and told me I had cancer. In that instant, I asked the universe, "Is this it? Is this going to take me out?" I very clearly heard in my head, "No." At that point, my journey and responsibility were to trust that higher voice, God's voice, and listen to what my American doctors had to say, but trust myself over what they had to say.

I've always known that you have to find your healing. When you are in a stress mode or experiencing chaos of any kind, your connection is less clear, and your guidance is less clear. Through it all, I know that I had to find what was going to heal me. The second time I had cancer, that understanding went a little deeper, a little farther, and it made my spiritual connection that much deeper.

I read a book called "Radical Remission" by Dr. Kelly Turner. That's when the light bulb went off. I had not dealt with my disease on any kind of an energetic level. I had done all the physical things that my integrative doctors told me to do. But, I hadn't addressed anything on a spiritual level or an emotional level. The energy work brought me deeper into the understanding that I was responsible for in my healing.

Energy work helped me through chemo, first of all. Then, I learned how to do energy work for myself. For three years, it kept me in a pretty good balance. I was cancer-free, healthy and happy, and doing all the "live in life." But then cancer returned. It's hard to understand this when you're in the throes of cancer. In hindsight, you're able to see the gifts that lie in the disease. It helped to bring me deeper into a spiritual connection. It helped me understand that I needed to tailor what I had learned a little bit more and pare it down and make it simple.

I was in pain for several months. I laid there thinking about love, praying and meditating. I feel like that was the turning point. The more I would try to heal cancer, the more my cancer grew. When I made the little shift to seeing myself as healthy and looking forward to things that I had yet to do in my life, I feel like that's when the shift occurred. I would meditate on love, all the people I love, all the love that was coming towards me, strangers that were sending me love, and above all, divine love. I could feel that love coming into my body, my energy body would light up, and I would revel.

It's such a comforting and soothing feeling to lay and revel in that feeling of unconditional love. I believe love is what does the healing. I knew the doctors would take care of the physical body, but I knew the emotional, energy and spirit bodies were my responsibility.

To me, that's the gift that's come out of the third time having cancer. I have much more appreciation for life and the beautiful little things that I took for granted. It can take a little while to get to that point where you see the beauty of what the disease has gifted you. There's trauma in it, but there is equally as much beauty, light, love and an enrichment of life.

When I got to Oasis of Hope, it was the first time that I talked with people who had cancer that had been healed by alternative treatments. Hearing personal stories at the hospital really gave me hope. This place is so accurately named. It is an Oasis of Hope. The hospital is totally different than any experience in the States. For me, it was the perfect fit. I believe that healing is mind, body, and spirit, and they address all of that here.

It's not just nutrition. I love all of the lectures that they have to offer here. There's no end to the educational components. I love that. I love how available the doctors are. You can just walk up and talk to them and the nurses. I have not met anyone who is not a delightful person, kind and committed to what they're doing here. That is refreshing.

Really, it's made me not want to go to a hospital in the States again. I just wish that this were available for everyone. I hope that people will at least call. I just say, call, and talk to somebody, and see what's possible. One visit here can make all the difference in whether you live or die, and the quality of your life.

—Anonymous

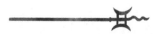

STORY OF HOPE

Paul Wyly • Embryonal Cell Carcinoma • 1975

In 1975, I was nineteen years old. A small painful nodule appeared on my testicle. After the testicle grew to about twice its normal size, I finally went to our doctor to check it. He referred me to a urologist, who immediately scheduled surgery to remove it.

The tests identified the malignancy as embryonal cell carcinoma. The doctor insisted on following up with major lymphatic surgery and chemo. "Without it, you only have two years," he stated. So I asked, "What are my chances if I have the surgery and chemo?" He told me that there was only a 30% chance of survival! I was devastated!

My father immediately began making calls and researching alternative treatment options. The Cancer Control Society put us in touch with the Contreras Clinic in Tijuana, Mexico, founded and operated by Dr. Ernesto Contreras, Sr. We left the hospital and started packing our bags.

As soon as we arrived at the clinic, they began lab work and removed my stitches. I began a regimen of laetrile, enzymes, and anticancer medication. They also put me on a strict diet of healthy foods. We attended seminars regarding health throughout our two-week stay at the clinic and went sightseeing most afternoons. We made new friends and had a wonderful time, which was great therapy in itself!

After returning home, I continued taking laetrile, enzymes, and anticancer medication. My mother faithfully prepared our meals from the laetrile diet, and I exercised regularly. I carefully avoided things that were unhealthy. After a few months, I noticed having a level of wellness and energy that I had not experienced since childhood. My outlook completely changed. I am now 64-years-old, am still healthy and eternally grateful to

God for the gift of hope and life given me all those years ago through the Contreras Hospital in Tijuana, Mexico!

After my experience, we have had several friends and family, who also received excellent results from the Contreras Clinic. When my wife was diagnosed in 2017 with breast cancer, there was no question where to go for treatment—Oasis of Hope Hospital! She is also doing very well! The Contreras family has indeed been a blessing to our family! It warms our hearts that Ernesto Contreras, Sr.'s legacy continues at Oasis of Hope Hospital, which is truly an OASIS OF HOPE! Thank you and may God continue to bless you all!"

—Paul Wyly
Hereford, Texas
United States

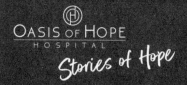

火攻

FOURTEEN

USE THE ELEMENTS

Those who use fire as an aid to the attack show intelligence;
those who use water as an aid to the attack
gain an accession of strength.

—Sun Tzu
The Art of War
The Attack By Fire

Hippocrates—the father of medicine—may be the most influential physician in history. He lived four hundred years before Christ, and thousands of years after his death, his observations and teachings continue to influence science and clinical practice. He was one of the first holistic physicians to treat a patient's body, mind and spirit. In other words, he practiced *wholism* (spelled with a "W," as in the word whole).

Hippocrates theorized that diseases were caused by an imbalance of a person and his relationship to his environment.

He defined health as a perfect balance between you and your environment. Hippocrates theorized that humans are composed of four humors, which are four different fluids— blood, phlegm, yellow bile and black bile. The balance between the humors determines whether a person is healthy or not. Hippocrates enriched his theory, known as *Humoral Medicine*, with the precepts of his Greek contemporaries Aristotle and Galen. He found a correlation between the four humors and Aristotle's basic elements that make up the matter on our planet —air, water, fire and earth (soil). Galen's four temperatures— hot, cold, moist and dry—became part of the overall theory too.[1]

Health is the perfect balance between humanity, the environment and God.

Faith Lagay, PhD articulates the correlation between Hippocrates' humors, Aristotle's elements and Galen's temperatures stating, "Blood was hot and wet like air; phlegm was cold and wet like water; yellow bile was hot and dry like fire; and black bile was cold and dry like earth."[2]

Hippocrates, and his contemporaries, were far ahead of their time. They theorized in an era before the technology existed that could confirm basic facts as simple as hemoglobin

being an oxygen-carrying vehicle. But, their intuition was right more often than wrong.

Hippocrates connected the four humors, elements, temperatures, and seasons to his patients' emotions and moods. From this arose the four personality types—Sanguine, Choleric, Melancholic and Phlegmatic. The moods associated with these personality types could change as a person would age, and with the seasons—winter, spring, summer and fall. If you study old school psychology, you will find that Sanguines are gregarious and generally optimistic. Cholerics tend to be pragmatic and easily angered. Phlegmatics have low levels of anxiety and depression. They like to go with the flow and avoid confrontation. Melancholics tend to suffer from anxiety more than others do.[3] Look at the table below, which organizes all of these aspects together.

Personality Type	Sanguine	Phlegmatic	Choleric	Melancholic
Humor	Blood	Phlegm	Yellow Bile	Black Bile
Element	Air	Water	Fire	Earth
Temperature	Hot & Moist	Cold & Moist	Hot & Dry	Cold & Dry
Age	Adolescence	Maturity	Childhood	Old Age
Season	Spring	Autumn	Summer	Winter
Organ	Heart	Brain	Gall Bladder	Spleen

Modern psychology frameworks for personalities, such as the Jung inspired Myers-Briggs model, have been used for occupational and relational satisfaction, and performance. These models could also be used as predictors of physical health. Many studies correlate personality types to mental health, and we see that, just as the ancient Greek physicians observed, the type could change over time. Current studies note that personalities tend to evolve to be more adaptive as a person grows older and matures.[4]

By embracing the interdependence of personality, emotions, moods and physical health, we find opportunities to enhance a patient's healing journey.

A HOLISTIC INFLUENCE ON MEDICINE AT OASIS OF HOPE

We find it striking that four hundred years before Christ, the Greek approach to medicine was integrating physical, emotional, seasonal, phase of life and personality types to help a person regain health. Hippocrates designed treatments integrating all of those factors. Back in the 1960s, our founder, Dr. Ernesto Contreras, Sr., took a an in-depth look at the Greek hospitals in the ancient era of Hippocrates. His eyes were opened and had an epiphany: A holistic model has greater potential to restore health than the reductionist model of 20th-century science and medicine.

Based on that awakening, he started to provide our patients with emotional and spiritual resources in addition to medicine for the body. We continue to do so more nearly sixty years after Dr. Ernesto Contreras, Sr. developed the Oasis of Hope *total care approach.*

In a strict sense, we do not practice humoral medicine. Our treatment goal is not balancing the humors of blood, phlegm, yellow bile and black bile. We are influenced, however, by the Greek humoral model as we design treatments for our patients.

Look at Oasis of Hope therapies through a lens of the four elements in the table below. We provide it as a visual, not scientific evidence.

Element	Therapies
Air	Ozone Autohemotherapy. Pentoxifylline.
Water	HDIVC. UVBI. Sodium Bicarbonate.
Fire	Hyperthermia.
Earth	Whole Food Plant-Based Nutrition. DCV. Mineral Replenishment Therapy. Nanoceuticals and Protein Supplement.

Our inspiration and treatment model has roots in ancient wisdom from the first century before Christ. We embrace the interlaced aspects of the body, mind, spirit and environment.

Even though the Greek physicians had very different religious beliefs than we do, they were seemingly in harmony with God's design. God has been embedded in the mind of every human, from Adam and Eve till now. His imprint on our soul is the intuition that tells us our bodies need balance. Natural elements provide the necessary sustenance to recuperate a healthy balance. That's at the core of the Oasis of Hope philosophy. When we break natural equilibriums, we lose our health. By restoring that balance, we can restore our health.

When provided with the right resources, the body will heal itself.

HOLISTIC VS. REDUCTIONIST

While I was traveling the world and producing the documentary series, *Healthy Long Life*,[5] I had the opportunity to interview Dr. Ramesh Chandra, the Chair of Chemistry at the University of Delhi. This university goes back to the British Raj and is home to a number of the first Nobel Prize Laureates for

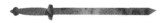

Chemistry. Dr. Chandra said that their research priority was to find the molecule, or the element, that will work to heal cancer.

After years of using the reductionist model, Dr. Chandra concluded that a single molecule could not provide a solution to cancer. He stated, "Reductionism doesn't work because the more we isolate elements and think we're getting closer, the less therapeutic the benefits we get." He said the answer to cancer would be holistic.

In another interview, T. Colin Campbell, Professor Emeritus of Cornell University, stated, "You can't do clinical trials on an apple." While many people say that clinical trials on non-patentable items, such as an apple, are not profitable, and therefore are not done, Dr. Campbell gave the real explanation. He shared, "The model for drug development is reductionist. If you're looking for the nutrient in an apple that cures arthritis, you will inevitably run into obstacles. Even if you find that nutrient that cures arthritis, when it's taken out from the rest of the apple, it loses its power because an apple has many different enzymes that make this nutrient work and activate synergy with the rest. Therefore, the healing power of food or whole food plant-based nutrition can never be studied conventionally because it has to work holistically." These interviews can be seen or heard on the Healthy Long Life documentary series.

We are encouraged by these comments from top university professors. Our therapies work synergistically within our holistic treatment model. Applying a reductionist model to our treatment approach would not be beneficial.

OASIS OF HOPE ELEMENTS

In this section of the book, we will explain how we employ nature's elements to undermine cancer. We do this as an integral part of our metabolic approach to cancer treatment. Each of the elements, present in a therapeutic form, acts on one or more of cancer's metabolic traits.

We love and use God-made cancer treatments like Ozone and whole food plant-based nutrition.

AIR

Air is made up of nitrogen, argon, helium and oxygen. Oxygen is especially essential to cancer treatment because hypoxia is a metabolic trait of cancer. Tumors thrive in an anaerobic environment. In other words, cancer grows stronger when oxygen levels are deficient. Healthy cells prosper in oxygen-rich environments. So let's talk about Ozone therapy again.

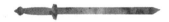

We especially appreciate Ozone therapy because it is a natural element created by God. Our bodies cannot live without oxygen. Oxygen is a gas made up of two atoms of oxygen and is denoted as O_2. Ozone is a gas made up of three oxygen atoms and is denoted at O_3. Our body thrives on oxygen, but Ozone must be treated with care because it can be toxic. If inhaled, it could result in lung damage. Fortunately, Ozone is non-toxic when administered via infusion, even at high dosages. I have infused myself with 60ccs of Ozone without any side effects. A positive side effect patients commonly experience is temporary euphoria. This occurs because Ozone therapy significantly increases oxygen levels. Let's explain how we administer Ozone at Oasis of Hope and its therapeutic benefits.

TARGETING HYPOXIA

Tumors are hypoxic because their aberrant vascular structure disturbs the microcirculation, which inhibits adequate cell respiration. Tumors are deficient at diffusing oxygen from malignant cell to malignant cell.[6] Hypoxia is strongly associated with tumor growth and spread, and it also makes cancer resistant to treatment. Hypoxia is a hallmark of cancer, and researchers have identified genes that are consistently affected by it. Recognizing the correlation between hypoxia scores and the impact on genes, scientists have assigned what they call *meta-gene signatures*.[7] A unique signature for many different types of tumors has been established based on each one's hypoxic status. The hypoxia status of a cell is an excellent diagnostic tool.

OXYGENATION IS KEY

A critical goal in cancer treatment is normoxia, a state of normal oxygen levels in malignant cells. Hypoxia generates the hypoxia-inducible transcription factor (HIF), which upregulates and downregulates over 100 genes.[8] HIF is one of the primary elements that causes malignant cell proliferation. Oxygen is needed for effective cancer treatment. A tumor's chaotic vascularization and poor microcirculation make it exceedingly difficult to deliver oxygen to malignant cells. Breathing pure oxygen does not affect cancer at all. But Ozone is a safe and effective means to restore normoxia in malignant cells. It will also unleash a cascade of other beneficial changes in a tumor's microenvironment. Though breathing pure oxygen does not affect tumors directly, there are a number of benefits for the immune system if the body can be in a highly oxygenated environment. Our hyperthermia machines are equipped with oxygen generators to create a high oxygen environment.

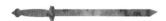

OZONE IS SAFE AND BENEFICIAL

Ozone therapy has been used medically for over one hundred years. When properly administered, it is safe and effective. It is an antibacterial, antiviral and antifungal.[9] It is also a potent immune stimulator. Opponents claim that oxygen therapies are "Expensive, unproven and harmful."[10] That could not be further from the truth. Oxygen is inexpensive and a readily available element. Ozone has been used safely in millions of people around the world, and benefits have been observed across the board. Clinical trials have concluded that Ozone administered in a medical setting does not cause any adverse effects, such as organ damage, and it does not increase mortality.[11]

INCREASING O_2 PARTIAL PRESSURE IN TUMORS

Researchers in Spain conducted a fascinating study with eighteen patients who had accessible metastases. The researchers were able to insert a probe into the metastatic tumor and measure the partial pressure of oxygen inside the mass. They assigned a hypoxia score based on the measurement. Remember, hypoxia is a significant factor that increases cancer growth and makes it resistant to treatment.

Once the oxygen levels were measured, each patient received Ozone Autohemotherapy (O₃AHT) three times on alternating days for just one week. At the end of the week, the partial pressure of oxygen was measured again. The result was that tumor hypoxia decreased in all of the participants.[12] Not one patient experienced any adverse effects. This clinical trial's results are paramount because the restoration of normoxia inhibits neoplastic growth and metastases.[13]

IMMUNE SYSTEM ACTIVATION & INFLAMMATORY RESPONSE SUPPRESSION

Ozone boosts the immune system by activating neutrophils and stimulating the production of cytokines. Cytokines send signals to immune cells that release a cascade of changes that help the immune system combat disease.[14]

As with many diseases, cancer activates the inflammatory response. Inflammation, in turn, helps cancer obtain more of the nutrients it needs to progress. One of the main culprits that provokes the inflammatory response is NF-κB. Studies have demonstrated that the mild oxidative stress induced by Ozone therapy will activate another nuclear transcriptional factor, Nrf2, which suppresses NF-κB. NF-κB suppression inhibits the inflammatory response, which helps cut tumors off from the nutrients they require to survive.[15]

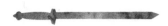

MECHANISM OF ACTION

Ozone (O_3) increases oxygen delivery to ischemic tissue and induces hydrogen peroxide (H_2O_2) formation.[16] O_3 is unstable and will react with any number of substances in the blood, including polyunsaturated fatty acids, ascorbic acid, uric acid and albumin. These compounds act as electron donors to O_3, and when combined, reactive oxygen species (ROS) and lipid oxidation products (LOP) are formed. In cancer treatment, the most critical ROS molecule is hydrogen peroxide (H_2O_2). When H_2O_2 is formed in the blood, it diffuses quickly into the cytoplasm, triggering numerous biological effects and stimulating multiple biochemical pathways. Several benefits are obtained, including a significant increase in adenosine triphosphate (ATP), which provides energy to cells and releases oxygen into malignant cells. Increasing oxygen levels in malignant cells makes them vulnerable to oxidative treatments such as High Dose Intravenous Vitamin C, chemotherapy and radiation.

OZONE AUTOHEMOTHERAPY (O_3AHT)

There are two viable means of increasing oxygen levels in tumors. As earlier established, breathing pure oxygen has no anticancer effect. But, if a patient breathes O_2 while under increased atmospheric pressure via a hyperbaric chamber, the partial pressure of O_2 will increase. Hyperbaric oxygen therapy (HBOT) provides numerous benefits to patients, but studies have shown that the increase in oxygen levels may dissipate in under fifteen minutes, whereas the increased oxygenation produced by Ozone autohemotherapy (O_3AHT) can last up to forty-eight hours.[17]

Oasis of Hope administers O_3AHT because it is the most effective way to oxygenate tumors and cause a cascade of therapeutic benefits. We draw two hundred milliliters of a patient's blood and introduce O_3 to the blood in a sterile container. Then the patient's ozonized blood is returned to the patient via a slow infusion. This therapy is well tolerated and valuable in cancer treatment because of the numerous positive biological and biochemical reactions it induces. As explained in a previous chapter, we utilize O_3AHT to increase the oxidative cancer-killing power of HDIVC.

BENEFITS OF OZONE THERAPY

We have been using Ozone for decades at Oasis of Hope. We have found it to be effective and safe. As with all therapies at Oasis of Hope, we go beyond our own observations and look to

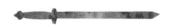

published data. According to numerous clinical studies, Ozone produces many benefits for cancer patients, including:

- Increased oxygen delivery to hypoxic tissues[18]
- Inhibition of growth of cancer cells[19]
- Inhibition of metastases[20]
- Induction of apoptosis in cancer cells[21]
- Decreased side effects from radiation therapy and chemotherapy[22]
- Improved therapeutic outcomes in patients undergoing radiotherapy[23]
- Lowered chemo-resistance in tumors[24]
- Protection of liver function[25]
- Help arrest hepatic dysfunction[26]
- Mitigation of rectal bleeding induced by radiation treatments in prostate cancer patients[27]

PENTOXIFYLLINE

The other therapy we categorize as an *air element*, is the vasodilator Pentoxifylline.[28] Hippocrates correlated the humor of blood to air. Hemoglobin delivers oxygen to every cell in the body. But a tumor's aberrant vascularization protects it from oxygen exposure. Pentoxifylline dilates blood vessels and facilitates better oxygen saturation levels within tumors.

Oasis of Hope employs Pentoxifylline to boost tumor oxygenation before and during HDVIC therapy. This drug is chiefly used to treat intermittent claudication, a condition in which poor blood flow to leg muscle leads to severe pain during walking. Pentoxifylline remedies this problem by improving blood flow to the legs.[29,30] It does so by exerting a range of effects that enable blood and red blood cells to flow through the microcirculation with less restriction. Pentoxifylline improves the flow of blood plasma by reducing blood viscosity. In part, this reflects lower blood levels of the protein fibrinogen, a significant contributor to blood viscosity. Pentoxifylline also makes the membranes of red blood cells and white blood cells more flexible, so that they can offer less resistance to flow as they pass through narrow capillaries.

By the same principle, Pentoxifylline therapy can make it easier for blood to flow through tumors. Tumor blood flow is often restricted because a tumor's vascular system tends to be chaotic and irregular.[31] Numerous rodent studies, and, to a more limited extent, clinical studies in humans, have shown that pre-treatment with Pentoxifylline can boost tumor blood flow and increase oxygen levels in poorly-oxygenated regions of a tumor.[32-48] These studies have been pursued primarily to make tumors more sensitive to radiotherapy, which is less effective at killing cancer cells in low-oxygen regions of tumors. Oasis of Hope has adapted this principle for use with HDIVC and O_3AHT. We have observed that this combination of therapies kills cancerous cells without harming healthy cells, and devastating the immune system, as do chemotherapy and radiation.

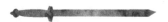

WATER

Another metabolic trait of cancer is that it thrives in an acidic environment. The extracellular fluid around tumors is acidic. As a tumor metabolizes glucose, it produces lactic acid. Oasis of Hope provides bottles of alkaline water to our patients, and we have alkaline water filling stations on every floor. According to clinical studies, drinking alkaline water with a pH near eight helps normalize intestinal health and supports a better night's rest.[49] But drinking alkaline water makes little contribution directly in the fight against cancer. When alkaline water is consumed, the gastric acid in the stomach neutralizes it before it affects tumors.

The most efficient way to interrupt lactic acidosis is by the administration of sodium bicarbonate.[50] More than ten years ago, clinical studies were conducted to measure the efficacy of intratumoral infusions of sodium bicarbonate. It was found that injecting tumors with baking soda was not more effective than taking it orally. We also found that drinking water with sodium bicarbonate mixed into water produced as good of a result as the expensive and uncomfortable procedure of injecting tumors directly.

There is clinical evidence that oral administration can be of benefit. A study on mice implanted with human breast cancer cells was conducted. The mice received a systematic daily dose of water with sodium bicarbonate. The results were that the progression of the growth of the primary tumor was slowed significantly, and the therapy minimized metastases.[51] Clinical studies have also demonstrated that hyperthermia increases the effect of decreasing the acidity of tumors.[52] Tumors brought into a neutral or slightly alkaline pH are less resistant to oxidative treatments. This is another great example of why we use combination therapies.

FIRE

Sun Tzu recognized that fire was the most potent weapon available to an army. We can see this in military terminology, in sports and pop culture. *Firepower* is defined as, "The capability of a military force, unit, or weapons system as measured by the amount of gunfire, number of missiles, etc., deliverable to a target." In sports, if a baseball player can throw very hard, sports commentators will say he can bring the *heat*. They may refer to a fastball as a *heater* when it crosses the plate at a higher than usual speed. A person is called a *fireball* when they are super energetic and never gets tired. The phrase *great balls of fire* was used in the 1800s to express the feeling of God's presence. Jerry Lee Lewis turned up the heat in the 1950s using the phrase to

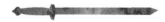

refer to the divine experience of the union between a man and a woman. A *heated* discussion is a very intense debate. Paris Hilton made *that's hot* a catchphrase people started using when they liked something. More recently, pop culture refers to anything that is extraordinarily great as *Fire*, as in, "Your new hairstyle is *fire*."

Since humans discovered how to make and control fire, it has been an essential resource because the human body cannot withstand extreme cold. Heat is also a potent anti-tumor agent. One of cancer's metabolic traits is that its cells cannot endure high core temperatures in the human body, as healthy cells can.

WHOLE-BODY HYPERTHERMIA

The *crown jewel* of Oasis of Hope's integrative cancer treatment is our unique whole-body hyperthermia protocol. Heating the core temperature of the whole body produces a tremendous anticancer effect and potentiates HDIVC. There are sound scientific reasons why these anticancer modalities interact synergistically.

Cancer researchers have made considerable strides in understanding how HDIVC can selectively cause cancer cell death while leaving healthy tissues unscathed. High dose infusions of Vitamin C can enter the blood and the tissue spaces between cells. Vitamin C donates an electron to molecular oxygen, which will generate the unstable free radical *superoxide*. Small amounts of extracellular free iron catalyze this reaction. Superoxide can't pass through cell membranes, but an extracellular enzyme called *superoxide dismutase* converts it to the compound *hydrogen peroxide* (H_2O_2). H_2O_2 readily passes through membranes.

Hydrogen peroxide can be lethal to all cells.[53] Healthy cells can tolerate higher levels of H_2O_2 than cancerous cells can. Healthy cells have sufficient levels of an enzyme called catalase, which converts H_2O_2 into harmless water. Malignant cells tend to have relatively low catalase levels, making them susceptible to death from H_2O_2-induced apoptosis.[54]

Hydrogen Peroxide is lethal to cancerous cells, but harmless to healthy cells.

Several years ago, researchers discovered that this wasn't the whole explanation. Even when cancerous cells had relatively normal catalase levels, they could be selectively killed by hydrogen peroxide. Researchers found that H_2O_2 is selectively lethal to tumors because cancerous cells generate high amounts of superoxide–the same compound that Vitamin

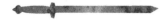

C can generate extracellularly. Malignant cells make more superoxide than healthy cells because via NADPH oxidase membrane complexes and their mitochondria.[55] When superoxide encounters hydrogen peroxide in the presence of small amounts of free iron or copper, it quickly reacts to generate hydroxyl radical.

Hydroxyl radical is a highly reactive biological compound. It can rip apart anything in its path, including membranes and the DNA vital for cell survival and growth. So when cancerous cells are exposed to high levels of extracellular Vitamin C, the hydrogen peroxide that flows into the cells encounters high levels of superoxide, leading to rampant production of hydroxyl radicals that can readily kill cancer cells.[56]

Hyperthermia induces apoptosis and potentiates oxidative therapies including HDIVC, chemotherapy and radiation.

So, how does the hyperthermia come into the picture? Cancer cells are selectively susceptible to killing by heat because the vascularization of tumors is aberrant, which doesn't allow them to dissipate heat the way healthy cells do. Clinical studies indicate that hyperthermia kills malignant cells by inducing apoptosis.[57, 58] However, whole-body hyperthermia alone rarely achieves substantial destruction of cancer cells, because the required level of sustained heat would be clinically intolerable. Humans can safely tolerate whole-body temperatures of 42°C (107.6°F) for several hours. That is usually not hot enough to kill a high proportion of cancerous cells. But using whole-body hyperthermia in combination with oxidative therapies like HDIVC, is a whole different proposition. Hyperthermia potentiates oxidative therapies including HDIVC, chemotherapy and radiation.[59]

One reason why heat is somewhat selectively toxic to cancer cells is that it boosts the production of superoxide by their mitochondria, which, as we have noted, is already notably higher in malignant cells. Scientists have demonstrated that bioengineering tumor cells with increased enzyme superoxide dismutase levels, in their mitochondria, protects them. The enzyme eliminates superoxide, and the cells are no longer so sensitive to killing by heat. Perhaps now you can see where our logic is going. Cancerous cells are selectively sensitive to the hydrogen peroxide generated within the tumor by HDIVC, in large part, because they make elevated levels of superoxide. Hyperthermia drives up the production of superoxide. Administering HDIVC right after hyperthermia generates a hydroxyl radical catastrophe for tumors.

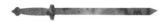

We reward our patients after hyperthermia with delicious-low glycemic index-organic-ice cold popsicles.

OASIS OF HOPE HYPERTHERMIA SYSTEM

The whole-body hyperthermia regimen we employ is effective and efficient. We have specialized hyperthermia pods that function has high-heat highly oxygenated cocoons. We provide each patient with an inner impermeable plastic suit to collect all of the perspiration, and an outer suit to trap heat. Our nurse assists our patients to get into the pod. We use the Oasis Oxy machine to saturate the pod with oxygen. The pod heats up rapidly and gradually increases the patient's core temperature to between 38°C and 42°C, and average temperature of 104°F. This therapeutic range of heat is reached in less than fifteen minutes. We maintain a patient's core temperature within that range for another thirty minutes. We follow the hyperthermia session with HDIVC and six grams of amygdalin.

We maintain optimal safety by continuously monitoring several clinical parameters, including core body temperature, oxygen saturation, blood pressure and pulse. An EKG is employed to detect heart arrhythmias should any develop. The pods close around the body, leaving the head outside and cooled by fans, which protects the brain from overheating. Many patients bring earphones and listen to relaxing music. When the session wraps up, we give a delicious, organic, low GI, popsicle that is lovingly made by our kitchen staff. Patients routinely tell us that a popsicle has never tasted as good that after a hyperthermia session.

The protocol is usually well-tolerated and does not damage healthy tissues–most notably, it doesn't damage the immune cells which toxic chemotherapies typically kill. Some patients report feeling light fatigue from heat exposure.

Hyperthermia is a powerful adjuvant therapy that we combine with our integrative therapies, including our whole food plant-based diet, HDIVC, nanoceuticals, amygdalin, emotional and spiritual support.

EARTH

For the element of earth, we take all of the healing medicine produced by God's pharmacy—vegetables, fruit, legumes, tubers, grains and seeds. Hippocrates said it best when he stated, "Let your food be your medicine and your medicine be your food." In the next chapter, we will expand on our Oasis of Hope nutritional therapy program.

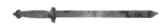

CONCLUSION

We use ancient Greek medical theories as our fundamental philosophy. We incorporate the most recent clinical data from medical journals to fortify our evidence-based holistic approach to cancer treatment. Once again, our focus is on improving your quality of life and extending the days you have on earth. We practice patient-centered, data-driven medicine that puts patients in the best position for their bodies to heal themselves.

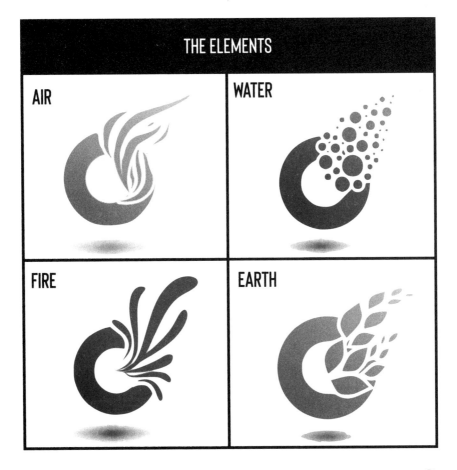

THE ELEMENTS

AIR

WATER

FIRE

EARTH

STORY OF HOPE

Bonnie Adolf • Stage IV Breast Cancer • 2016

My journey began in the spring of 2016 when I received the news that my latest mammogram showed something suspicious. That's when the sky fell. The diagnosis was stage 4 breast cancer. I was whisked off to see an oncologist where immediate chemo treatments began. Everything happened so fast. Treatments began, awful side effects, loss of hair, weigh loss, no appetite at all, lethargic most of the time. After six months of chemo, I was told that nothing had improved, and in fact, my tumors had grown! All I could do at that time was cry. I was given one more heavy-duty treatment and told to reach out to the groups that do clinical trials.

At the end of my three weeks at home, and getting through that last treatment, I knew I could not continue to live like that. I called my doctor and told her I would not be returning. Then the most miraculous thing happened. Friends brought a book titled *Where the Amish go for Cancer Treatment*. That's where I learned about the Oasis of Hope in Mexico. After reading, I knew I wanted to go. We called, they said come, and off we went on our miraculous journey! The greatest thing for me was that my husband was included in my room and board and was with me throughout the entire time.

We received a warm welcome and settled in our room. Then treatments began. They were all non-invasive, and the setting was absolutely comforting. I loved the soft music. We were blessed with many new friendships while there.

The greatest blessing was the news from Dr. Contreras that all cancer was gone, except for the primary tumor in my breast. After being discharged, the recommendation was to see my breast surgeon on our way home. We left Mexico on Thursday afternoon, and on Saturday morning I was in surgery. What a journey!!!

Oasis of Hope was a wonderful place to be and experience the most excellent care and treatments. It was all so very different from the treatment I had received where I live.

Praise Jesus!! Today I am going on four years cancer-free and feeling like a new person. I'm loving life and spending time with family and friends. My only regret is that I did not know about Oasis of Hope before I started chemo treatments.

I'm so thankful for the nutrition classes and lectures that have taught me how to make the changes that have kept me healthy and changed my life. To the doctors and staff of Oasis of Hope, my most sincere gratitude for all you have done for me. I tell everyone about you. Blessings to you all!

–Bonnie Adolf
Show Low, Arizona
United States

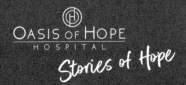

用間

FIFTEEN

BE VIGILANT

*What enables the wise sovereign and the good general
to strike and conquer, and achieve things
beyond the reach of ordinary men,
Is foreknowledge.*

—Sun Tzu
The Art of War
The Use of Spies

General Sun Tzu, was one of history's wisest military strategist. He used spies to continually monitor the enemy as a strategy to diminish the loss of troops. Those charged with keeping a watchful eye on their enemy's movements have been important to the security of every nation, body of people and tribe since the earliest civilizations. Songs have been written about essential personnel like the watchmen of ancient Israel.

All Along The Watchtower is a part of many of our live's soundtrack.[1] Jimi Hendrix recorded the song on the *Jimi*

Hendrix Experience Electric Ladyland album in 1968.[2] Hendrix' cover of the Bob Dylan masterpiece rocketed into the Rock 'N' Roll cosmos, landing it at #47 on *Rolling Stone Magazine*'s definitive list of the 500 greatest songs of all time.[3]

All Along The Watchtower
(Excerpt)
by Bob Dylan

All along the watchtower
Princes kept the view.
While all the women came and went
Barefoot servants too
Outside, in the distance
A wildcat did growl
Two riders were approaching
The wind began to howl.

People often search for deeper meaning in the song's words that emanated from Dylan's soul. Is *All Along The Watchtower* spiritual or mystical? Is it Biblical or psychedelic? The world may never know, but it's plausible that the lyrics' inclusion of a watchtower, a prince and a pair of horseback riders could be referencing the Lord's Word given to the people of Israel through the great prophet Isaiah.

Prepare the table, watch in the watchtower, eat and drink.
*Arise, you **princes**, and oil the shields. For thus the Lord has said to me: "Go,*
*station a **watchman**; let him declare what he sees.*
*When he sees chariots with **horsemen in pairs**, a chariot of donkeys,*
and a chariot of camels, then let him pay close attention,
very close attention." Then the watchman called:
"O Lord, I stand continually on the watchtower in the daytime,
and I am stationed at my guard post every night. Look, here comes a chariot
of men, horsemen in pairs."
And he answered and said, "Fallen, fallen is Babylon.
And all the graven images of her gods lie shattered on the ground."[4]

—Isaiah 21:5-9

In the ancient city of Jerusalem, guards were posted to watchtowers. They were to be vigilant, watch for any threat and sound the alarm when danger was approaching. God also posted spiritual watchmen, prophets like Isaiah and Jeremiah. They were vigilant and sounded warnings against the spiritual threats that would take down the nation. Unfortunately, Israel often did not heed the warnings. They would turn away from God and let the enemy waltz right in and conquer their cities. God's people paid the price for not being vigilant in prayer, and vigilant in monitoring the movement of enemy troops. At Oasis of Hope, we try to help our patients be vigilant so they won't pay the price of being taken by surprise by a cancer recurrence.

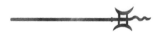

VIGILANCE IS MANDATORY

When fighting cancer, vigilance is of paramount importance. We have to continually watch and observe a patient to make sure that cancer does not spread. Even when metastases occur, being vigilant helps us detect them early. Early detection is critical in every stage of the evolution of cancer.

In this chapter, we will share how to be vigilant. We will also explain how we, as your treatment partners, will be vigilant against a recurrence and the spread of cancer to other organs. This chapter discusses the strategies, therapies, and activities a patient can do to prevent cancer. We will talk about healthy changes in diet and lifestyle. We will encourage you to make healthy choices and avoid returning to bad habits that work against healing, such as smoking or alcohol consumption.

OASIS OF HOPE VIGILANCE TOOLBOX
Medical Evaluations • Lab & Imaging Tests • Nutrition
Emotional Support • Patient Education & Empowerment
5-Year Follow-Up Program

In the previous chapter, we spoke extensively about recurrence, and how a strategic plan of attack must include therapies to minimize the risk of cancer coming back stronger.

Our focus on vigilance is to defend against recurrence and metastases. Let's go through our vigilance toolbox.

MEDICAL EVALUATION, LABORATORY TESTS & IMAGING

As your treatment partners, we will be vigilant through medical evaluations, both at the hospital and by phone when you are back home. In addition to consultations, we will utilize laboratory tests and imaging studies such as PET scans, CT scans, X-rays and ultrasounds. Before we explain more about these studies, let me warn you about the emotional toll it can take if you base your hope on the numbers and results of such studies.

EMOTIONAL ROLLERCOASTER

Imagine having four children going through the teenage years at the same time. Social pressures are so high these days, chances are, at least one of the four will have some distressing situation going on at any given moment. I remember a day many years ago, when my four teenagers were in tears at the same time. The crying was contagious but I resisted joining in. I had learned that it doesn't inspire confidence in children for a father to join them on the ups and downs of an emotional rollercoaster.

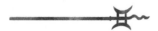

What helps is for a dad and mom to keep it steady. Kids can tether themselves to their even-keeled parents and feel safe.

In the cancer journey, there are emotional rollercoasters that are tempting to get on. A consultation with a doctor to review tumor markers and radiology reports can be one such rollercoaster. If the report comes back showing improvement, a person can go to an emotional high. Later, if an oncologist shares a report indicating that cancer is progressing, emotions can plunge back down. I recommend keeping emotions down-to-earth and regarding medical evaluations, lab tests and radiological studies for what they are—medical tools that help doctors and patients be vigilant about the care that is needed.

MEDICAL EVALUATIONS

A competent physician does not make medical decisions solely by the numbers. Laboratory results and radiology reports may indicate the treatment is taking the patient toward the goal of long-term survival with a high quality of life. But much of the data in such reports can mean something different depending on other factors. Therefore, a good doctor may gain insights through speaking with the patient that lab tests cannot reveal. Suffice it to say, you are more than numbers on a piece of paper. Your health needs and condition are complex and cannot always be detected through lab tests. A doctor's experience and intuition are key elements to helping you on your health journey.

**Tether your emotions to God's Word,
not a doctor's words.**

LABORATORY TESTS

Laboratory tests use samples of a patient's blood, urine or other bodily fluids. These tests are used for diagnosis, staging, treatment planning, monitoring progress, identifying oncogenes, identifying tumor specific antigens and detecting metastases or cancer recurrence. They are also used to determine a person's overall health and functioning of the immune system.

Tests include blood chemistry, complete blood count, cancer gene mutation testing, cytogenetic analysis, sputum culture, immunophenotyping, tumor markers and urinalysis.[5] You need to understand that these tests, no matter how sophisticated they may be, are not definitive and cannot be looked at with a one hundred percent confidence level. Results vary from person to person, and more importantly, results can vary for the same patient from day to day. A person's lab numbers can change due

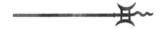

to what has been eaten, the occurrence of a non-cancer-related illness such as a cold, medications and other factors. Instead, of basing your outlook on the ever-changing numbers, work with your doctor who will interpret the true meaning of the tests within the context of your general health, your treatment response and evolution.

IMAGING

Have you ever looked at a CT scan image or ultrasound and tried to figure out what is being revealed? Radiologists study and practice for years to learn how to interpret what they are looking at and provide a diagnosis. But, looking at images to make a diagnosis is like looking at tea leaves to come to an accurate understanding of your destiny. Interpreting radiology studies is less of a science, and more of an art.

Many studies have been published about the error and discrepancy rates of radiologists' performances. Such studies have found an error rate of up to twenty percent in all studies combined. Diagnosis of breast cancer through mammography has a sixty-one percent rate of error. The error rate of cancer CT studies is thirty-seven percent.[6]

Radiological studies are incredibly valuable in the diagnosis and evaluation processes. They help doctors keep vigilant and look for early warning signs of recurrence and metastases. But, considering the average error rate in the interpretation of images, we encourage you not to ride the radiological report rollercoaster. Medical evaluations, laboratory tests and imaging studies are useful tools. But, they don't conclusively determine the probability of life extension and the quality of life you can enjoy throughout your healing journey. They are tools that help us in our vigilance, nothing more, nothing less.

A VICTOR'S MENTALITY

In the previous section, we showed how a patient's emotions could be influenced by lab tests and radiological studies doctors use to be vigilant against cancer. Now, we want to talk about how you can be emotionally vigilant against a victim's mentality. Seeing yourself as a cancer victim promotes negative emotions that suppress the immune system.

It is common for patients to feel that they were dealt a bad hand in life when they were diagnosed with cancer. Our counselors work closely with patients to encourage them, and show them how to transition from a cancer victim to a cancer victor.

It's helpful to become aware of the emotional stages you have experienced from the moment you were diagnosed until

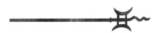

now. Self-awareness is the first step to developing a cancer victor's mentality. One of the best explanations of these stages is in the Warner Brothers' film *The Bucket List*, starring Jack Nicholson and Morgan Freeman. The plot is about two cancer patients, Edward (Nicholson) and Carter (Freeman), who in normal life would never associate with each other. They meet at a hospital where they are both being treated for cancer. They bond over the shared experience, and a friendship ignites. Edward suggests that Carter write out a list of all the things he would like to do before kicking the bucket, hence the name *The Bucket List*.

In a memorable scene, Edward and Carter are walking down a hospital corridor with their IV poles, and Edward asks if Carter had heard about the stages of grief cancer patients go through when they are diagnosed and treated. Since Carter hadn't, Edward goes through an in-depth explanation of the stages of denial, anger, depression, bargaining, and the final stage—acceptance. Carter, impressed by Edward's knowledge of the stages, asked, "So which stage are you in?" "**Denia**l," replied Edward.[7]

His response provided an unforgettable moment of comic relief while making an important point. You may have filled your brain with useful information. Still, it is up to you to act on the acquired knowledge and develop a mentality that will move you forward, and get you unstuck from denial, anger, depression or bargaining. A cancer victim can be detected when people get stuck, and are not moving forward through the stages. A cancer victor can be identified because they have moved to the stage of acceptance.

Surrender to the sovereignty of God brings deep peace, bolsters hope and provides the power to push through the difficulties on the cancer journey.

David Kessler and Elisabeth Kübler-Ross, the developers of the five stages of grief, make a clarifying point about acceptance. Acceptance is not being ok with what has happened, or what is taking place. It's not throwing in the towel. Acceptance is learning how to live with your circumstances and resolving to move forward the best way you can.[8] Once you accept what's happening, you can resolve to take action. Resolve is apparent in people that can say, "It's cancer. It's real, and I'm going to do everything within my power to live and enjoy my life to the fullest."

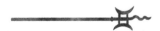

As the great psychiatrist Viktor Frankl taught that you cannot control everything that happens to you. You can control how you choose to react to a situation.[9] Resolve drives the determination to do everything in your power to extend your life, improve its quality, trust God and accept whatever the outcome of your effort is. Surrender to the sovereignty of God brings deep peace, bolsters hope and provides the power to drive you through the difficult cancer journey. Acceptance, resolve and surrender are essential traits of a cancer victor mentality. They are the foundation of power, determination and grit.

THE POWER OF THE PLATE

Once you resolve to be a cancer victor, you will discover that there are many tools at your disposal. Food choices may be the most potent tool in your toolbox. Dr. Scott Stoll is the doctor who coined the term "Plantrician," which means a physician who uses whole food plant-based nutrition as medicine. He points out that everyday people sit down to eat three meals a day, which translates into taking an average of one hundred bites daily. Because of the frequent, constant repetition, the power of the plate has the most potential to transform your life and get you headed toward full healing.[10] Leveraging the power of the plate means making healthy food choices. That sets you up on a platform for success.

**Plantrician: A physician who uses
whole food plant-based nutrition as medicine.**

It is disheartening to witness patients start to experience significant improvements, only to backslide to old lifestyles and lose all of their gains. One of our goals is to help our patients enjoy life while being vigilant against old bad habits. We continuously motivate our patients to be good stewards of their healing. We understand that recipes must be delicious for people to choose healing foods over the harmful deep-fried, highly salted, high-fat, low-fiber mainstays of the SAD (Standard American Diet) diet. We share our tantalizing and delectable recipes available on our nutrition blog and clean eating cooking app for all to enjoy.

In 2013, we interviewed fifty of our long-term cancer victors. We were looking for the success factors that helped them beat cancer. Forty-eight of the fifty victors cited faith and food. Imagine how important the power of the plate is considering that ninety-six percent of our cancer victors listed food as one of the most critical factors to undermining and overcoming cancer. We were so impressed with our cancer victors that we published their comments in our book *50 Critical Cancer Answers*.[11]

Faith and food are essential to healing.

FOOD NOURISHES YOUR SOUL

We strongly believe that food choice is the most potent and effective tool against cancer in the long-term. Food works at the molecular level. It can upregulate or downregulate gene expression. It works through cell signal transduction, and can cut off the supply line to cancer if the right food is consumed. But food doesn't only work on the body, it also nourishes the soul.

Food is a powerful way to communicate to the sub-conscious. Each time you make a food choice, you send a message, either positive or negative, to your psyche. You may, or may not, realize that we communicate with ourselves continuously. Sending mixed messages is counterproductive. A mixed message would be like choosing to eat a hamburger, fries, and milkshake after you finished taking a cancer-fighting therapy. Taking valuable treatments tells your body that you care about it, and you are determined to nurture it back to health. Eating unhealthy foods tells your body you don't care about it and are willing to abuse it. So which message is your body to believe? Do you care about your health or not?

Making healthy food choices is healing self-talk that nourishes the soul. But doing something harmful is telling your body that you don't love it, and this brings the human spirit down. Imagine saying, "I have cancer, I'm going to commit to this therapy and do it," followed by, "I'm going to have a smoke." Your subconscious will question, "What is it? Are you trying to heal me, or are you trying to kill me?" These types of mixed messages are devastating to the immune system.

LOVE YOUR BODY & SOUL AS YOU LOVE YOURSELF

The power of the plate is at your disposal. Healthy food choices send a clear message to your body and nourish your soul. Every time you say, "I am not going to have fried chicken strips, but I'm going to eat this whole food plant-based meal," you tell your body that you care. When you choose healing foods at each meal and snack time, you provide your body with the nutrients it needs to heal, and send your soul the powerful message, "I'm sacrificing my cravings because I love you."

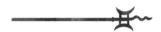

Self-love will help you be vigilant against a cancer recurrence or spread. A cancer victor is love-driven to do everything necessary to slow, control and reverse cancer when possible. A cancer victim is fear-driven, which is not helpful. Cancer victors have thoughts like, "I'm doing the right things because it keeps me healthy, and I am caring for my body." On the other hand, cancer victims have thoughts like, "I am going to do these things because the cancer is going to come back, and if I don't do it, the cancer is coming back." Developing a cancer victor's mindset is vital for healing and essential to remain vigilant.

MORE MIXED MESSAGES

We talked about how a patient can send mixed messages by eating right and still smoking. Equally as counterproductive are the mixed messages sent by oncologists. Contradicting messages frequently arise around the topic of nutrition. We witnessed this first hand while visiting a top cancer treatment center in Jakarta, Indonesia.

The thirty-seven-story cancer center was equipped with three PET scans. It was luxurious and boasted the best oncology care in the region. While we were amazed by the technology and architecture, the oncologists wanted to hear how we use whole food plant-based nutrition as a part of our therapy. We shared how many of our patients told us that when they asked their oncologists what they should eat, inevitably, their doctors told them that it didn't matter as long as they kept their caloric intake up to avoid muscle wasting. Many oncologists recommend milkshakes because of the high caloric value. Why would an oncologist recommend a sugary drink when sugar feeds cancer? Considering that these oncologists prescribe chemotherapy, and chemotherapy really upsets the stomach, they ignorantly tell patients to eat or drink whatever they can tolerate and not throw back up. We assume they must not know better if they don't help patients wield the power of the plate! We teach our patients how to manage adverse side effects with healing foods. For example, we recommend drinking ginger tea to calm the stomach and make way for nutritious food.

One oncologist at the center in Jakarta shared a patient story with us. His testimony underlined that what a doctor recommends for nutrition can send an unintended message to a patient. The doctor's patient asked what she needed to be eating. He gave the standard oncology answer that it didn't matter what she eats. The doctor explained that she should eat whatever she could hold down, but the patient went home thinking, "It doesn't matter what I eat because I'm going to die."

Two weeks later, the patient's son returned extremely worried because his mother had completely stopped eating. The oncologist asked why the patient stopped eating, and the son replied that his mother saw no point because the doctor said she was going to die. The oncologist exclaimed that he never said that. Still, the patient interpreted the message, "It doesn't matter what you eat," to mean, "Eat whatever because you are about to die."

It could be that oncologists in the US are limited to phrases and messages approved by corporate lawyers. Suggesting anything beyond FDA approved chemotherapy, could get an oncologist in legal hot water. An oncologist is expected to prescribe FDA approved oncology medications. Food is not an FDA approved drug, so an oncologist will be reluctant to talk about food. If a patient is fortunate, the oncologist may refer them to a nutritionist. But many nutritionists prescribe high caloric diets void of whole food plant-based nutrition.

TEXTBOOK ONCOLOGY

Using food as medicine is absolutely not a part of any oncology textbook. If an oncologist were to speak about the healing power of food, they would risk receiving negative peer pressure. Once we met an open-minded oncologist in Newport

Beach who told us, "If you want textbook results, then provide textbook chemotherapies. If you aren't happy with textbook results, you have to give the patient much more. Otherwise, they are at risk." At Oasis of Hope, we want better than textbook results, so we teach about healing foods and alternatives no matter what peer-pressure we may receive from conventional oncologists.

HOW YOU SAY IT MATTERS

Sometimes it's not the message, but how it's presented. For example, if you went to a food truck to order a veggie taco plate with a hibiscus, it may cost $6 to $8. If you order a similar veggie taco plate at *True Food Kitchen*, it will likely set you back $12 plus another $5 for a sweet infused water. Though the food may be similar tasting, the price is higher at the restaurant because of the artful presentation, service and ambiance. Presentation is a difference-maker. The way a physician presents information affects a patient's desire to fight. If a patient has a poor prognosis, the wrong way to share the difficult news is to say, "You will die in three months if you don't start chemo. With treatment, you could live up to a year." There is some dishonesty in that presentation, though the oncologist may not be aware. One problem with the statement is that an oncologist does not know for certain if the patient will die in three months without chemotherapy, or if chemotherapy could extend the patient's life beyond that timeframe. Statistics are for reference, but they are not definitive for a patient.

An honest and compassionate way to communicate the message of a poor prognosis would be to say, "The cancer is at an advanced stage, and it is going to be a tough fight. But I am ready to do everything I can to help you live longer and have the best quality of life possible. Considering your condition, I need you to commit to doing everything you can to help me help you. If we work together, and do everything we know how to do, you may beat the statistics. But for sure, you will have a better quality of life for however long you live." This honest, clear messaging can inspire a patient to fight.

**Fight the good fight,
and leave the results up to God.**

Messaging is a vital factor in the treatment of patients. Presenting information in a hopeful way will often produce better results. But, other oncologists push back against such messaging. Once, at a conference I was speaking at, an oncologist accused me of giving false hope. I informed him that there is no such thing as true hope or false hope. Either there is hope, or there isn't hope. Taking away hope from a patient, by focusing on negative statistics, or by telling them it doesn't matter what they eat, is not compassionate and it's unethical. Statistics are there to help us understand the level of vigilance we must apply. Statistics are there to help us understand the level of vigilance we must apply. But, statistics do not determine a patient's treatment outcome.

Oasis of Hope holistic therapies elevate the patient and undermine cancer's strongholds.

No matter what textbook statistics say, we work hard with our patients to get better results. Our holistic approach is based on nourishing the body and soul, boosting the immune system and applying our multi-pronged strategy. It elevates the patient and undermines the strongholds of cancer. When a patient is willing to make all of the necessary lifestyle changes, and the treatment center has conventional and alternative medicine available, there is hope. To date, we have not discovered a cure for cancer. We don't have a cure. We don't advertise or promise a cure. What we have is good medicine, and we partner with our patients for life. Together, our doctors and patients fight the good fight and leave the results up to God.

PATIENT EMPOWERMENT

Fighting cancer cannot be a passive activity. A patient cannot go to an oncologist and say, "Fix me," and expect the doctor to order treatment, a nurse to infuse chemotherapy and sit back waiting to be healed. Your body is not a car, the hospital is not a repair shop, and the doctor is not a mechanic. You must lead your fight against cancer.

Imagine that your dream was to summit Mount Everest. You would probably look for a *Sherpa* to help you reach your goal. A Sherpa is a member of the Himalayan people living on the borders of Nepal and Tibet, renowned for their mountaineering skills.[12] Foreigners hire Sherpas for their knowledge and experience of climbing Everest. But even if you found the best Sherpa, you couldn't expect to tell him, "Carry me to the top."

No one can summit Everest for you. Summiting the highest mountain in the world is more about the fight to get there, than reaching the top. Though the effort must come from the climber, nobody can summit Everest alone. Let's apply this to the fight against cancer. In this analogy, you are the climber, Everest is cancer, and your doctor is the Sherpa that will provide the necessary knowledge, equipment and sundries for climbing the mountain. The Sherpa cannot guarantee summiting Everest, but he can go every step of the way with the climber and provide guidance based on his countless years of experience.

As your treatment partners, we are committed to going every step of the way with you, and providing guidance based on our fifty-seven-plus years of treating tens of thousands of patients. We will give you the needed resources, but you have to bring the fight. Oasis of Hope is structured to provide resources to our patients' bodies, mind and spirit. We want to share a bit more about these resources, which can serve as tools for your vigilance against cancer.

EDUCATION IS KEY

Accurate information applied correctly is powerful. We don't only treat our patients, we educate them. Each day, we have a different presenter to speak about therapies, nutrition, emotional healing and home therapy. Patient empowerment is one of our goals. Through education, we can help develop a patient's ability to be vigilant against cancer.

CELL SIGNALING TRANSDUCTION

One of the things we do during lectures is to ask patients to visualize what can happen to a malignant cell with the administration of specific nutrients. We explain how specific nutrients work against cancer and travel through pathways in the body to complete assigned tasks. Education on nutrition is vital because the nutrients in food have healing power. Eating the right foods is the easiest way for patients to be proactive and vigilant against the advance of cancer.

Nutrients work against cancer via cell signaling transduction. Cells stay in a healthy balance through constant communication (cell signaling) with each other. Depending on what nutrients are put into the body, the transduction of signals can either promote cell life or cell death. Many studies identify nutrients in fruits, vegetables and tubers, that act on multiple signal transductions that induce apoptosis—programmed cell death—in cancer cells.[13] Some of the most important anticancer nutrients are curcumin (the active nutrient in turmeric), EGCG, genistein, silymarin and resveratrol. They affect inflammatory responses, growth factors, transcription factors and protein kinases.[14]

When there is a malfunction in cell signaling, it can affect various physiological processes. It can result in inducing harmful conditions such as massive insulin resistance, glucose intolerance and tumorgenesis.[15] Whole food plant-based nutrition promotes homeostasis and empowers the immune system to be vigilant against malignant cells.

How can we leverage the power of cell signaling against cancer? We can answer the question with one word–nutrients. With the right nutrients circulating throughout your body, cell signaling and immune response will function properly. Promoting an optimal functioning immune system is paramount because there is no greater anticancer agent than your God-given defenses.

Clinical studies have identified a number of metabolic routes that malignant cells depend on. Studies have also identified nutrients that can cause cell signaling that is detrimental to the survival of cancerous cells. We use nutrients, such as the ECGC in green tea, to target cell signaling in cancer cells' metabolic routes. The nutrients can inhibit or kill the cells.

We educate our patients on the anticancer power of nutrients to help them see beyond the food on their plate or a handful of capsules. We believe that this knowledge will inspire people to keep on our nutrition program and be less anxious about having to maintain a supplementation routine we prescribe. Instead of thinking about wanting to eat unhealthy food, we invite our patients to visualize the nutrients from healthy foods going into their bodies with the assignment of seeking and destroying cancer cells.

**There is no greater anticancer agent
than your God-given defenses.**

A war analogy could be useful to visualize the effects of anticancer nutrients. Imagine that we are using nutrients to cut off communication to malignant cells. In war, if you bomb the opposition's radio tower, they will be rendered incapable of doing anything. Or if you destroy railways, then the opposition will be unable to move their essential supplies.

Alternatively, imagine your enemy is driving along a high and curvy mountain road, which has a tall cliff on one side and a steep ravine on the other. Traffic signs are essential to guide a driver through a precarious route. In this story, you've been tasked with taking the enemy out, but you do not have any weapons. One way of harming the enemy without firepower is changing the road signs. Imagine that the sign warns of an upcoming sharp turn to the right, but you change it to indicate that the turn is to the left. The enemy will drive off the cliff because of the sign change. Nutrients have this sign-changing potential along cancer's metabolic pathways.

TARGETING CANCEROUS CELLS

Let's connect your food choices to cell signaling that targets cancerous cells. Insulin Growth Factor (IGF-1) increases the risk of proliferation of several cancers such as breast, colorectal, lung and prostate.[16] IGF-1 is associated with the oncogenic process, which is a threat, but also an opportunity. The opportunity is to reduce the serum levels of IGF-1 by eating the way we teach at Oasis of Hope. According to a large clinical study conducted by Cancer Research UK, lower levels of total IGF-1 are associated with a plant-based diet.[17]

There is an essential amino acid called methionine, which is abundant in animal proteins from a meat-based diet. Too much methionine can shorten our lifespans. Our chief researcher, Mark McCarty, had a study published that stated, "Plant proteins—especially those derived from legumes or nuts—tend to be lower in methionine than animal proteins. Furthermore, the total protein content of vegan diets, as a function of calorie content, tends to be lower than that of omnivore diets, and plant protein has somewhat lower bioavailability than animal protein. Whole food vegan diets that moderate bean and soy

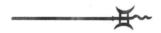

intake, while including ample amounts of fruit and wine or beer, can be quite low in methionine, while supplying abundant nutrition for health. Furthermore, low-fat vegan diets, coupled with exercise training, can be expected to promote longevity by decreasing systemic levels of insulin and free IGF-I."[18] Now that is the scientific power of the plate!

IT'S DELICIOUS!

Honestly, the food at Oasis of Hope is delicious. Under the direction of our nutritionist Rosa Contreras-Tessada, we have a culinary team that works hand in hand with our medical department to ensure that we provide delectable foods that have the therapeutic nutrients we wish to promote. Cooking is an art our team has mastered. We share recipes and cooking skills with our patients. The whole food plant-based diet at Oasis of Hope is the only delicious cancer treatment we have ever encountered. We have an executive chef who is an expert in vegan food. Together with our culinary team, he ensures the food is delightful to the taste buds. The main dishes' presentations are a feast for the eyes as well. We just love gathering our patients around our round tables to make new friends and enjoy a hearty healing meal three times a day. People feel loved by the way our team plates up and serves the food. The highlight of each week is a special menu and entertainment at mealtime on Wednesdays. Oasis of Hope meals are a food fiesta!

Oasis of Hope serves up delicious healing foods straight from its rooftop garden.

We understand that it can be a big ask of people to trade in steak and potatoes for veggie lasagna and cucumber water. But it is our joy to show the incredible variety of the healing foods God put on earth, and share how delicious the food is when fresh and prepared right. We are aware that food preparation can be a big challenge once a patient returns home. But maintaining the Oasis of Hope diet is one of the most important keys to being vigilant against the progression of cancer. So, we empower our patients through food prep classes.

WHERE THE MAGIC HAPPENS

We have culinary magicians in our kitchen, but our training bar for our patients is where the real magic happens. Our teaching chef gives cooking classes to our patients and their loved ones. The recipes are posted on our nutrition blog and

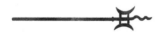

app. We have utensils for each person sitting at the bar, and as chef demonstrates how to prepare one of our delicious dishes, everyone can cook along. It is a time of joy, laughter and unity— three ingredients that boost the immune system. We teach food safety and knife skills that are necessary to prepare the whole food recipes right. We do all we can to impart knowledge and skills to help our patients continue a healthy lifestyle after they leave the hospital.

FROM ROOFTOP TO TABLE

Surely you have heard the phrase, "From farm to table." It is said that it doesn't get fresher than that. Well, we beg to differ. We grow much of our produce right at the hospital on our rooftop garden. We are obsessed with producing nutrient-rich, pesticide-free organic produce to the point that we prepare our soil. We have a team member that goes through the labor-intensive process of organic composting. Composting is great for the environment and producing the highest quality of organic microgreens, green leafy vegetables, herbs and a seasonal selection of vegetables and fruit.

On occasion, we get our patients involved in the growing processes. If we are ready to plant, we can invite our patients to get their hands in the dirt. Working with soil is profoundly therapeutic. It's especially impacting when a patient can plant, pick, produce, and prepare a plate of delicious food at our training bar. Yes, that is why that place where magic happens at Oasis of Hope is our food prep training bar.

Not everyone wants to cook. We get it. Some patients opt for sitting in on the sessions to enjoy tasting and get their fill of the great information our teaching chef imparts. That is fine by us. But, when you come to Oasis of Hope, try cooking with us. You are sure to love it!

POWER OF THE PLATE IN YOUR POCKET

Our nutritionist Rosa, our teaching chef and the kitchen studio crew work hard every week to put the power of the plate in your pocket. When we say, "Put in your pocket," we are not talking the way little children try to hide icky vegetables in their pockets! We are talking about our recipe app that can be downloaded to the phone you keep in your pocket.

We invite our patients to download our app cooking called *Healthy Long Life*. It's available for free on the Apple app store or Google play. It is ideal for anyone who wants easy to prepare healthy vegan recipes. It puts recipes for breakfast, lunch, dinner, side dishes, sauces, and desserts right at your fingertips. Each recipe has instructions and a sixty-second high-speed cooking demonstration video. The video shows the ingredients, utensils and appliances needed to prepare each dish. A picture paints one thousand words, so we decided to show how to cook each recipe. We do all we can to make things simple.

The app's shopping list is another cool feature. If you see a recipe you like, you can touch the shopping list icon, and the ingredients populate the shopping list. When you go to the grocery shop, you can pull it up the list. As you pick up each ingredient at the store, you can cross the item off on the list. When you are done shopping, you can delete the list.

Connecting with the earth, and the food it produces resonates with the body, mind and spirit.

TREATMENT COMPLIANCE

As you started reading this chapter, you saw that the topic was vigilance against cancer progression and spread. But then, the chapter started talking about medical consultations, laboratory and radiology tests, and food. The purpose was to be practical and share with you the tools we use, and you will need to use to be vigilant. We provide these resources to empower you to get and stay healthy.

Positive caring messages, a healthy diet and regular evaluations are determining factors for a long-term victory over cancer. But there is one factor that is the absolute most important one.

Treatment compliance is the most significant way to protect against a cancer recurrence and metastases.

Many years ago, a naturopathic doctor, named William Crawford, referred seven patients to us. Dr. Crawford had a private practice in North Carolina. That same year, a vitamin salesperson out of Atlanta, Georgia, also sent us seven patients. Reviewing our records, we found that all seven patients referred by Dr. Crawford were alive after five years later. Only three of the seven patients referred by the vitamin salesperson were still alive.

We decided to investigate to find out what the difference-maker was. We contacted Dr. Crawford and asked what treatments he was administering to the patients he had referred to Oasis of Hope. He told us that he didn't change any of the Oasis of Hope protocols. We asked him what he thought was behind the high rate of survival of his patients. He thought it was our therapies. But, we knew it was more than that because the other group of patients had not faired as well. We asked him to be specific about what he was doing with his patients, and he told us that he would have them come in a minimum of once a year for an evaluation. Also, he would call them a few times a year to encourage them to keep on the Oasis of Hope protocol, even if it was just continuing to eat a whole food plant-based diet.

We received terrific feedback from Dr. Crawford, but we still needed to find out what may have contributed to the lower survival rates from the patients referred to us by the vitamin salesperson. We were stunned by her attitude. She almost wouldn't talk to us, stating, "I will never refer a patient to you again." We asked what she did to support the patients after they returned from Oasis of Hope. She had continued to sell her vitamins to them. We asked if she had encouraged the patients to continue on the medications, supplements and diet we had prescribed, and she said that she had not.

The answer to long-term survival was staring us right in the face. The most important thing to be vigilant about is treatment compliance. Do the program and continue to do the program. When we researched the medical literature, we found that we were really on to something. A study conducted with ninety-four cancer patients measured the effect treatment compliance had on survival rates. In the study, several factors were measured that could increase survival. The study concluded that three factors contributed to more prolonged survival—how severe the cancer was, compliance with treatment, and being involved in a support program.[19] Many other studies conclude that treatment adherence is associated with longer survival rates in all types of cancer including lung, pancreatic, prostate, colon, ovary and breast.[20]

We saw we had an incredible opportunity to help our patients live longer and enjoy a higher quality of life. Dr. Crawford had intuitively been doing the right things. He had been educating his patients on our protocols, and about the value of strictly adhering to our treatments. He implored them to not abandon or deviate from the treatment just because they were feeling good. Understanding that treatment compliance and encouragement were the difference makers led us to an important realization. Most of our patients do not have a Dr. Crawford in their hometown. They don't have anyone that can teach and encourage them about Oasis of Hope therapies. It was up to us to structure an aftercare program where we could keep a patient informed, and encouraged to continue the treatment and healthy lifestyle changes they had made. That is why Oasis of Hope care extends beyond the walls of our hospital.

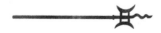

OASIS OF HOPE FIVE-YEAR FOLLOW-UP PROGRAM

At Oasis of Hope, we want to be your partner for life. *Partners For Life*, refers to the **purpose** and **duration** of our partnership with you. The purpose we share with each patient is to help them add years and quality to their lives. The duration of the relationship is for the rest of our (patients and doctors) lives.

Because the first five years are the most critical in the battle against cancer, we developed and implemented a five-year program. We are proactive instead of reactive. We don't wait for a patient to call us when they need us. We are vigilant with our patients, and at the time of discharge, we get follow-up calls on our calendar for the next five years. Every day, our computer pulls up the calendar, and our follow-up coordinators make calls to patients all around the world. Their objectives are to encourage treatment compliance and educate as necessary. Some of the calls are just to check in with our patients. Other calls are actual medical consultations with the doctors. Follow-up calls give us more opportunities for evaluation. Sometimes our doctors make adjustments to protocols. Other times, they request new lab work or radiology tests. Sometimes they determine that it would be beneficial for the patient to come for additional treatment at the hospital.

Because treatment compliance is the most critical factor for vigilance against cancer, we put our money where our mouth is. How? We don't charge our patients for our five-year follow-up program. We provide five years of calls for encouragement, counsel and re-evaluation absolutely free of charge.

This close contact allows patients to clear up any doubts about their prescriptions. We can encourage them to keep on the regimen. There are times when patients need our counsel to get emergency care. By being in constant contact with our patients, and supporting them in their aftercare, we send an important message—they are never alone when going through the cancer journey.

CANCER STEM CELLS

One of the reasons why cancer recurrence is frequent is that even when a tumor is destroyed, cancer stem cells generate chemoresistant malignant cells.[21] Researchers don't know how or where cancer stem cells originate, and until recently, no viable therapy against them was available. Fortunately, an off-label use of a diabetes drug has demonstrated its ability to control cancer stem cells. The drug is affordable and readily available.

Oasis of Hope uses an affordable and effective drug to inhibit cancer stem cells.

Metformin, a drug whose structure was based on the bioactive compounds in the traditional anti-diabetic herb Galega Officinalis ("goat's rue"), is currently the most prescribed agent worldwide for control of type 2 diabetes. Its efficacy in this regard appears to reflect its ability to activate an enzyme known as AMP-activated protein kinase (AMPK).[22,23] AMPK functions as a kind of cellular fuel gauge, becoming activated and signaling when the high-energy catalyst ATP is in short supply. AMPK causes cells to burn more fuel to generate ATP while suppressing non-essential cellular activities that use ATP. In the liver of people with diabetes, AMPK spares ATP by slowing the rate at which liver cells produce and release glucose. One of the reasons diabetics' blood sugar levels are chronically high is that their livers consistently produce elevated levels. Metformin, via AMPK activation, slows the rate at which the liver releases glucose, and this is thought to be the chief way in which it is helpful in diabetics.[24]

Now, what about Metformin and cancer? Interest in Metformin as an agent for preventing and controlling cancer was triggered by epidemiological studies examining cancer rates in diabetics. Diabetics tend to be more cancer-prone than non-diabetics, and that have poorer prognoses when they get cancer. However, studies found that diabetics treated with Metformin, compared with diabetics treated with other drugs, were less likely to develop several types of cancer–breast, prostate, colon, lung, and pancreatic, hepatic among them.[25-37] Moreover, when researchers focused on diabetics who already had cancer, in many studies, though not all, they found that the those taking Metformin had longer survivals than the ones not taking it.[34,38-44]

A key to Metformin's ability to prevent and restrain cancer is its capacity to inhibit the enzyme complex *mammalian target of rapamycin complex 1* (mTORC1). mTORC1 is chronically activated in most cancers. This complex causes cancerous cells to increase their production of proteins that boost cellular proliferation, enable cells to invade surrounding tissues, and evoke new blood vessels that feed the tumor (angiogenesis). It also prevents apoptosis, the cell-suicide mechanism.[45] Apoptosis helps prevent cancers by killing off pre-cancerous cells that have sustained damage to their DNA. It also is the chief mechanism whereby chemotherapy and radiotherapy kill cancer cells. mTORC1 activity promotes cancer growth and shields cancer from chemotherapy.[45] As a

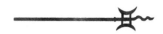

mTORC1 antagonist, Metformin is a valuable cancer prevention and control agent. These findings gave rise to multiple studies in which immunodeficient mice implanted with various human tumors were treated with Metformin. In many though not all of these studies, Metformin was found to slow cancer growth.[46-62] Other studies examined the interaction of Metformin with chemotherapy or radiotherapy in animal tumor models. Many of these studies found that chemotherapy and radiotherapy were more effective for killing tumor cells and restraining cancer growth when Metformin was co-administered.[47,54,63-69]

While Metformin's ability to potentiate conventional oncology treatments is partially attributable to an inhibition of mTORC1 via boosting cellular capacity for apoptosis, it is now clear that this phenomenon also reflects Metformin's ability to increase the vulnerability of cancer stem cells to therapy. Cancer stem cells (CSCs) are a small subpopulation found in tumors that tend to be extraordinarily resistant to killing by chemotherapy, radiotherapy, and hyperthermia.[70] CSCs can proliferate and give rise to all cancer cell types needed for a tumor to grow and spread. So killing CSCs is imperative in cancer therapy. For reasons not entirely understood by science, Metformin can kill or prevent the formation of CSCs and slow their growth.[71-89] Metformin sensitizes these cells to killing by chemotherapy, radiotherapy and hyperthermia.[47,71,73,75,84,90,91] Remember, hyperthermia is a highly effective part of the oncology protocols at Oasis of Hope.

Oasis of Hope—Tomorrow's medicine today.

In light of these provocative findings, numerous clinical trials worldwide are in progress in which Metformin, alone or as an adjuvant to other cancer-killing measures, is being tested in patients with a variety of cancer types. Within several years, there will be sufficient data to explain Metformin's anticancer mechanisms. At that time, more oncologists may wake up to the benefits and start prescribing it to their patients. It won't surprise you to learn that Metformin has already been in use at Oasis of Hope for many years, in line with the dictum: *tomorrow's medicine today*. We leverage Metformin as an adjuvant to out unique therapeutic strategy that combines HDIVC with whole-body hyperthermia and other therapeutic agents.[92]

One of the cancer-promoting proteins whose synthesis is boosted by mTORC1 is *hypoxia-inducible factor 1alpha* (HIF-1alpha). This protein is rapidly degraded when cells are

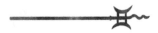

well oxygenated, but it has a prolonged half-life in oxygen-deprived tumor regions. HIF-1alpha helps cancer cells to survive, grow and spread in the low oxygen environments that tumors often encounter.[93] Another effect of HIF-1alpha activity is to render cancer cells more resistant to killing by high external concentrations of ascorbate.[94] Though cancer cell lines are readily susceptible to killing by Vitamin C in oxygenated cell cultures, tumors in animals or patients are not as responsive to IV Vitamin C in comparable concentrations.[95,96] Oasis of Hope's strategy for overcoming this effect is to decrease tumor levels of HIF-1alpha. We do this with a two-fold approach: 1) Decreasing tumor synthesis of this protein by administering Metformin, and 2) Promoting its degradation by boosting tumor oxygenation with the drug Pentoxifylline.

A recent study with human breast and pancreatic cancer cell lines revealed that Metformin may have a complementary, or synergistic, interaction with hyperthermia in the killing of cancerous cells and CSCs.[84] This study also determined that hyperthermia ,of the magnitude employed at Oasis of Hope activates AMPK and suppresses mTORC1, which is complementary to the impact of Metformin in this regard.

In doses typically prescribed for diabetes, Metformin is a very safe and inexpensive drug. It does not produce any of the characteristic toxicities of cytotoxic chemotherapies, and it does not depress the bone marrow. Its chief side effect, affecting a small percentage of patients, is gastrointestinal upset. When this problem presents, it can often be managed by starting with a lower dose of Metformin, and gradually increasing it. In addition to its utility in diabetes and cancer therapy, Metformin can benefit health in several ways, including longevity and anti-aging.[97-99]

CONCLUSION

We are thrilled that you have invested in your health by educating yourself with this book. It is our honor to present the knowledge and strategies we have developed and refined over the last six decades. Through the chapters, we shared about the history of Oasis of Hope and our founder, Dr. Ernesto Contreras, Sr., because his treatment philosophy determined the trajectory of the way we treat our patients and the protocols that we develop. We explained how cancer can be treated effectively as a metabolic disease and how cancer's metabolic traits can be used against it. We went through the shortcomings of chemotherapy and radiation, and the effective way to use conventional therapies supported by alternative therapies. Then, we laid out our multipronged treatment strategy that leverages cancer's

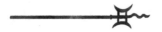

strengths and weaknesses to overcome threats and take advantage of the opportunities to weaken and destroy cancer. We explained our *Core* and *Enhanced* therapies that serve to kick the legs out from under cancer while restoring the best cancer-fighter known to humankind—your immune system. We talked about the different interventions we use to minimize and be vigilant against the spread and recurrence of cancer, including controlling cancer stem cells. In this final chapter, we shared how we commit ourselves to our patients for life through our follow-up program.

The Oasis of Hope Total Care Approach is *The Art & Science of Undermining Cancer*

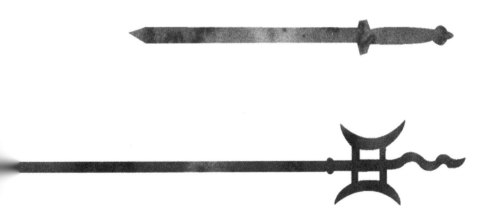

YOU ARE THE CENTER OF ALL OF OUR EFFORTS

The only reason Oasis of Hope exists is to help you. Oasis of Hope will do all that is possible. Our main objectives are to:

- Inspire a victor's mentality extend life for as long as **possible**
- Maintain the best quality of life **possible**
- Do all that is **possible**
- Trust God to do the im**possible**

This holistic, comprehensive treatment approach is

The Art & Science of Undermining Cancer.

Do all that is possible. Trust God to do the impossible.

But Jesus looked at them and said,
"With men this is impossible,
but with God all things are possible."

—Matthew 19:26 MEV

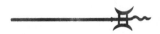

STORY OF HOPE

May Orr • Stage III Breast Cancer • 2003

I was diagnosed with stage three breast cancer after I found a lump that was 2.5cm x 1.5cm. This happened in November 2003 and was quickly followed by my first visit to Oasis of Hope in January 2004.

The oncologist in the U.K. wanted to start me on chemotherapy and hormonal treatment ASAP, as I was sixty years old at the time. Having always used alternative treatments for any ailment that I had up to that point, and seeing the effect that conventional chemotherapy had on other people, I wanted to see what other options were available to me before I signed up for anything.

Having found out about Oasis of Hope through a family friend, and knowing at that point they were solely doing alternative treatments, I decided that I would be better off there and would take my chances, bearing in mind that there were no guarantees. Of course, I had some reservations, like having to travel all the way to Mexico and having to pay a lot of money for my treatment, instead of being treated for free in the U.K.

Within a day of arriving at the hospital, my nerves and fears were quickly allayed, and I knew that I was at the right place. All of the treatments were clearly explained. The staff was very friendly and helpful. Even though my only prior experience of being in the hospital was giving birth to my two children, the atmosphere at Oasis of Hope was unlike any other hospital that I had ever been in or visited.

My body adapted very well to the treatments and, due to the distance that I had to travel each time, I was able to spread out my visits to every six months, which then became annual visits after five Years, and I remained in remission for nearly fifteen years. Blessings.

—May Orr
Edinburgh
Scotland

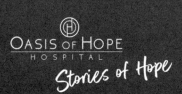

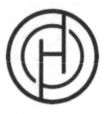

CONCLUSION

In 2003, our founder, (father, grandfather) graduated to heaven. It was forty years after he, and his wife Rita, opened the Oasis of Hope Hospital. It has been our privilege to continue his healing legacy. We know that people facing cancer have many options to choose from when selecting a treatment center. We are not the perfect fit for everyone. But, for those who are drawn to us; to those looking for combination therapies that bolster the immune system, minimize side effects and champion a patient's quality of life—for those people, we are here for you. It is our honor to be your healing partner for life.

Dr. Contreras, Sr. taught us that all healing is the work of God. Our purpose is to provide resources to the whole person—body, mind and spirit—to give a patient's body the best opportunity to heal itself, and protect itself from a recurrence of cancer. Our treatment strategies slow cancer for some patients. In other cases, it controls cancer. In a number of cases, it completely reverses cancer and takes it into full remission. No matter what the objective results are, we know that nearly all of our patients experience favorable subjective results. What are subjective results? We see that most of our patients suffer less side effects, have an increase in energy, experience a decrease in pain and feel much better with Oasis of Hope treatments than they did taking conventional therapy.

Dr. Contreras, Sr. also taught us the healing power of love. He loved his patients like his own children. We continue in this spirit of love, though we won't go as far as the *Beatles* did when they sang, "All we need is love." But, we know that love is an essential part of treatment, and it's powerful when added to a combination of therapies.

A doctor who loves his patient like he loves his wife, children and mother, will infuse hope and peace to his patients. When a patient has an increase in peace, and a decrease in fear, the immune system gets stronger. We could make a scientific case on how love is an immune building emotion, but instead, let us just loving our patients is just part of the Oasis of Hope DNA.

Oasis of Hope began with God's love for patients that He impressed in Dr. Ernesto Contreras, Sr.'s heart. He paraphrased the Bible's love chapter to apply to his profession as a medical doctor.

1st Corinthians 13
Paraphrased for Physicians
by Dr. Ernesto Contreras, Sr.

"Though I become a famous scientist or practicing physician,
and I display in my office many diplomas and degrees,
and I am considered as an excellent teacher or convincing speaker,
but have no love...
I am just a sounding brass or tinkling cymbal.
And though I have the gift of being an exceptional clinician
making the most difficult of diagnoses;
and understand all the mysteries of the human body;
and feel sure I can treat any kind of disease, even cancer,
but have no love...
I am nobody.
And though I invest all my money to build the best facilities,
buy the best equipment, have the most prominent physicians
for the sake of my patients;
and I devote all my time for their care,
even to the point of neglecting my own family or myself,
but have not love...
it profiteth me nothing.

Love is an excellent medicine.
It is non-toxic;
it does not depress the body's defense,
but enhances it.
It can be combined with all kinds of remedies,
acting as a wonderful positive catalyst.
It relieves pain and maintains
quality of life at its best level.
It is tolerated by anyone;
never causes allergies or intolerance.

Common medicines come and go.
What was considered good yesterday,
is useless now.

What is considered good now,
will be worthless tomorrow.
But love has passed all tests and will be effective always.

We now know things only partially,
and most therapies are only experimental.
But when all things are understood,
we will recognize the value of love.
It is the only agent capable of creating good rapport
between patients, relatives and doctors,
so everybody will not act as children,
but as mature people.

Today, many truths appear as blurred images to us as physicians,
and we can't understand how the things of the spirit work to maintain life;
but one day we will see all things very clearly.

And now these three basic medications remain:
Faith, hope and love.
But the greatest of these is love."

Dr. Ernesto Contreras, Sr.'s love for his patients was inspiring. The fuel to the Oasis of Hope mission is:

Sharing the healing power of faith, hope and love.

It is our joy, privilege and honor to love each patient that is drawn to Oasis of Hope. Who knows? Maybe you will be our next story of hope!

STORY OF HOPE

Linda Brown • Stage II Breast Cancer • 2014

Just before Christmas of 2014, I was diagnosed with breast cancer, stage 2 ductal carcinoma, with lymph node involvement. My local oncologist prescribed the traditional treatments consisting of months of chemotherapy, radiation and eventually surgery. While I was never given a definitive prognosis, my oncologist considered it a serious matter. After a few days of shock, I knew I needed a plan of care that aligned with my belief system. Being a chiropractor for over twenty-five years, I favor alternative treatments that support innate healing when possible. I do not avoid traditional care when necessary, but look for a more balanced approach.

I remembered, from years prior, that a friend told me about Oasis of Hope. I started my research. What I found was an approach to cancer that was perfect for me. Oasis of Hope offered a balanced approach to cancer treatment offering alternative and traditional methods based on individual cases. Its survival rate for breast cancer was up to five times better than traditional treatment alone.

Within a few weeks, I was at Oasis of Hope for treatment. Immediately the staff of doctors and nurses eased all of my fears. I could sense that I was in the right place for my healing. I underwent the prescribed metabolic treatment protocols as well as surgery and immunology. Three months later, my PET scan showed no evidence of disease! I continued to be cancer-free for five years until a recent new episode of breast cancer. My only thought at the new diagnosis was how fast I could get back to Oasis of Hope! I returned "Home" to Oasis of Hope early in 2020, and started treatment again. I am pleased to report that I had my checkup in July, 2020. The mammogram and ultrasound showed no sign of disease—praises to God and Oasis of Hope.

When friends ask me why I chose Oasis of Hope, I tell them not only do they have cutting edge cancer treatments, they also treat the whole person, and not just their disease. Supporting every aspect, including spiritual and mental health, is an essential part of healing at Oasis of Hope. I highly recommend Oasis of Hope!

—Linda Brown
Lynchburg, Virginia
United States

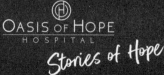

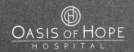

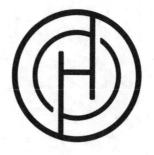

ABOUT THE AUTHORS

Francisco Contreras, MD serves as the general director and chairman of the Oasis of Hope Hospital. He is the son of the Oasis of Hope Hospital founder, Dr. Ernesto Contreras, Sr. He has been treating cancer patients for the last thirty-seven years. Dr. Contreras is recognized worldwide as an authority on integrating alternative cancer treatment with conventional medicine. He has been a guest on Fox and Friends, CNN, MSNBC, DayStar, CBN, Univision and Telemundo. He has been featured in many documentaries, including *The Truth About Cancer*, and he was a medical consultant for the movie *Letters to God*.

Dr. Contreras completed his pre-med in Pasadena, California, medical school in Toluca, Mexico, and his specialty in surgical oncology at the University of Vienna in Austria, where he graduated with honors. Dr. Contreras has authored and co-authored numerous books about health and integrative therapy including, *50 Critical Cancer Answers, The Hope of Living Cancer Free, The Coming Cancer Cure, Beating Cancer* and *Dismantling Cancer.*

Daniel E. Kennedy is a psycho-oncology counselor who has served as chief executive officer and vice-chair of Oasis of Hope Hospital since 1993. He is the first grandson of Dr. Ernesto Contreras, Sr. For the last twenty-seven years, he has counseled and ministered to patients. His three master's degrees are in counseling, ministry and business. He is an ordained minister in the Wesleyan Church.

As a part of Daniel's mission to help people prevent and reverse illness, he has met with, and interviewed, some of the world's top researchers at the World Health Organization, the Max Planck Institute, Cancer Research UK, McGill University, the University of Shizuoka, Beijing University, the University of Delhi and the Institute for Genetic and Biomedical Research in Sardinia. The interviews can be seen in the documentary series *Healthy Long Life.*

www.HealthyLongLife.com

ACKNOWLEDGMENTS

All healing is of God. Works that foster the love of God and humankind have eternal significance. These two truths were ever-present throughout the research and writing of this book.

We would like to thank our wives, families, patients, the entire Oasis of Hope team, Rosa Contreras-Tessada, Marcela Contreras-Santini, Dr. Francisco Ceceña, Dr. Paulina Lárraga and Mary Bernal. We also wish to thank our applied nutritionist and phenomenal researcher—Mark McCarty. Oasis of Hope owes much of its advances to Mark's tireless research.

NOTE TO THE READER

The Art & Science of Undermining Cancer was co-written but often speaks in the first person and expresses the opinions and experiences of Dr. Francisco Contreras, Daniel E. Kennedy, or both, although they are not individually identified throughout the book. All testimonials submitted by Oasis of Hope cancer victors are included in this book with their consent.

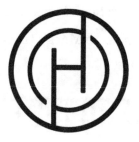

REFERENCES

CHAPTER 1

1. Rosenthal, E., & Plunkert, D. (n.d.). How health insurance changed from protecting patients to seeking profit. Retrieved from https://stanmed.stanford.edu/2017spring/how-health-insurance-changed-from-protecting-patients-to-seeking-profit.html

2. D'Agostino, J. (1976, November 05). Ernesto Contreras' TJ laetrile clinic. Retrieved from https://www.sandiegoreader.com/news/1976/nov/04/cover-cancer-connection/#

3. Pear, R. (1986, November 15). Reagan signs bill on drug exports and payment for vaccine injuries. Retrieved from https://www.nytimes.com/1986/11/15/us/reagan-signs-bill-on-drug-exports-and-payment-for-vaccine-injuries.html

4. Laetrile Report Under Fire From Within. Science News, 00368423, 1/7/1978, Vol. 113, Issue 1

5. Mouaffak Y, Zegzouti F, Younous S, et al. Cyanide poisoning after bitter almond ingestion. Annals of Tropical Medicine & Public Health [serial online]. November 2013;6(6):679-680.

6. Luque-Almagro, V. M., Cabello, P., Sáez, L. P., Olaya-Abril, A., Moreno-Vivián, C., & Roldán, M. D. (2018). Exploring anaerobic environments for cyanide and cyano-derivatives microbial degradation. Applied Microbiology and Biotechnology,102(3), 1067-1074. doi:10.1007/s00253-017-8678-6

7. Moss, R. Second Opinion. http://www.secondopinionfilm.com/wp-content/uploads/2014/01/anatomy_of_a_coverup_so_02.pdf]

8. National Cancer Institute. Laetrile/Amygdalin (PDQ®) Overview. http://www.cancer.gov/about-cancer/treatment/cam/patient/laetrile-pdq#section/_3

9. Makarević J, Rutz J, Blaheta R, et al. Amygdalin Influences Bladder Cancer Cell Adhesion and Invasion In Vitro. Plos ONE [serial online]. October 2014;9(10):1-11.

10. Sireesha D, Reddy BS, Reginal BA, Samantha M, Kamal F. Effect of amygdalin on oral cancer cell line: An in vitro study. Journal of Oral Maxillofac Pathol 2019: 23:104-7

11. Yang C, Zhao J, Cheng Y, Li X, Rong J. Bioactivity-guided fractionation identifies amygdalin as a potent neurotrophic agent from herbal medicine Semen Persicae extract. Biomed Research International [serial online]. 2014;2014:306857.

12. Mirmiranpour H, Khaghani S, Esteghamati A, et al. Amygdalin inhibits angiogenesis in the cultured endothelial cells of diabetic rats. Indian Journal of Pathology & Microbiology [serial online]. April 2012;55(2):211-214.

13. Yang H, Chang H, Kim C, et al. Amygdalin suppresses lipopolysaccharide-induced expressions of cyclooxygenase-2 and inducible nitric oxide synthase in mouse BV2 microglial cells. Neurological Research [serial online]. 2007;29 Suppl 1:S59-S64.

14. Zhu H, Chang L, Li W, Liu H. Effect of amygdalin on the proliferation of hyperoxia-exposed type II alveolar epithelial cells isolated from premature rat. Journal Of Huazhong University of Science and Technology. Medical Sciences = Hua Zhong Ke Ji Da Xue Xue Bao. Yi Xue Ying De Wen Ban = Huazhong Keji Daxue Xuebao. Yixue Yingdewen Ban [serial online]. 2004;24(3):223-225.

15. Chang HK, Shin MS, Yang HY, Lee JW, Kim YS, Lee MH, et al. Amygdalin induces apoptosis through regulation of Bax and Bcl-2 expressions in human DU145 and LNCaP prostate cancer cells. Biol Pharm Bull 2006;29:1597-602.

16. Chen Y, Ma J, Wang F, Hu J, Cui A, Wei C, et al. Amygdalin induces apoptosis in human cervical cancer cell line HeLa cells. Immunopharmacol Immunotoxicol 2013;35:43-51.

17. Yang C, Li X, Rong J. Amygdalin isolated from Semen Persicae (Tao Ren) extracts induces the expression of follistatin in HepG2 and C2C12 cell lines. Chin Med 2014;9:23.

18. Qian L, Xie B, Wang Y, Qian J. Amygdalin-mediated inhibition of non-small cell lung cancer cell invasion in vitro. Int J Clin Exp Pathol 2015;8:5363-70.

19. Park HJ, Yoon SH, Han LS, Zheng LT, Jung KH, Uhm YK, et al. Amygdalin inhibits genes related to cell cycle in SNU-C4 human colon cancer cells. World J Gastroenterol 2005;11:5156-61.

CHAPTER 2

1. Shilliday, B. (2018, June 14). Angelina Jolie's Ex-Husband Billy Bob Thornton Says Those Necklaces Weren't 'Buckets Of Blood'. Retrieved from https://hollywoodlife.com/2018/06/13/angelina-jolie-billy-bob-thornton-blood-vial-necklaces-explained-smear/

2. Marsden, S. (2013, May 14). Angelina Jolie: I had a double mastectomy to reduce my breast cancer risk. Retrieved from https://www.telegraph.co.uk/news/celebritynews/10055488/Angelina-Jolie-I-had-a-double-mastectomy-to-reduce-my-breast-cancer-risk.html

3. Pitt, A. J. (2015, March 24). Angelina Jolie Pitt: Diary of a Surgery. Retrieved from https://www.nytimes.com/2015/03/24/opinion/angelina-jolie-pitt-diary-of-a-surgery.html

4. https://www.nytimes.com/2015/03/25/science/experts-back-angelina-jolie-pitt-in-choices-for-cancer-prevention.html?action=click&module=RelatedCoverage&pgtype=Article&region=Footer

5. BRCA Mutations: Cancer Risk & Genetic Testing. (n.d.). Retrieved from https://www.cancer.gov/about-cancer/causes-prevention/genetics/brca-fact-sheet

6. John, E. M., Miron, A., Gong, G., Phipps, A. I., Felberg, A., Li, F. P., ... Whittemore, A. S. (2007). Prevalence of pathogenic BRCA1 mutation carriers in 5 US racial/ethnic groups. JAMA, 298(24), 2869–2876. Retrieved from http://search.ebscohost.com/login.aspx?direct=true&AuthType=shib&db=mdc&AN=18159056&site=eds-live&scope=site

7. Chong, H. K., Wang, T., Lu, H.-M., Seidler, S., Lu, H., Keiles, S., Elliott, A. M. (2014). The validation and clinical implementation of BRCAplus: a comprehensive high-risk breast cancer diagnostic assay. Plos One, 9(5), e97408. https://doi.org/10.1371/journal.pone.0097408

8. What Is Cancer? (n.d.). Retrieved from https://www.cancer.gov/about-cancer/understanding/what-is-cancer#how-cancer-arises

9. NCI Dictionary of Cancer Terms. (n.d.). Retrieved from https://www.cancer.gov/publications/dictionaries/cancer-terms/def/neoplasia

10. Are Stem Cells Involved in Cancer? (n.d.). Retrieved from https://stemcells.nih.gov/info/Regenerative_Medicine/2006chapter9.htm

11. Kim, S. (2018, January). Cancer Energy Metabolism: Shutting Power off Cancer Factory. Retrieved from https://www.ncbi.nlm.nih.gov/pmc/articles/PMC5746036/

12. Givant-Horwitz, V., Davidson, B., & Reich, R. (2005, June 01). Laminin-induced signaling in tumor cells. Retrieved from https://www.ncbi.nlm.nih.gov/pubmed/15890231

13. Gatch, W. D. (1957, May 01). Degree of Cohesion of Cancer Cells and Its Relation to Cancer Spread. Retrieved from https://jamanetwork.com/journals/jamasurgery/article-abstract/554993

14. Too much DNA: A new way to target cancer cells? (2016, January 08). Retrieved from https://uwmadscience.news.wisc.edu/basic-science/too-much-dna-a-new-way-to-target-cancer-cells/

15. Wishart, D. S. Is Cancer a Genetic Disease or a Metabolic Disease? EBioMedicine 2015 June; 2(6): 478-479.

16. Yan, L., Rosen, N., & Arteaga, C. (2011, January). Targeted cancer therapies. Retrieved from https://www.ncbi.nlm.nih.gov/pmc/articles/PMC4012258/

17. Nci, Nci, & Nci. (n.d.). Addressing Cancer Drug Costs and Value. Retrieved from https://www.cancer.gov/news-events/cancer-currents-blog/2018/presidents-cancer-panel-drug-prices

18. Davios, K. (2018). In Developing Payment Mechanisms of Gene Therapies, the US Has a Long Road Ahead. AJMC. Retrieved from https://www.ajmc.com/focus-of-the-week/in-developing-payment-mechanisms-for-gene-therapies-the-us-has-a-long-road-ahead

19. Jones, W., & Bianchi, K. (2015). Aerobic glycolysis: beyond proliferation. Frontiers in immunology, 6, 227. doi:10.3389/fimmu.2015.00227

20. Iansante, V., Choy, P. M., Fung, S. W., Liu, Y., Chai, J. G., Dyson, J., ... Papa, S. (2015). PARP14 promotes the Warburg effect in hepatocellular carcinoma by inhibiting JNK1-dependent PKM2 phosphorylation and activation. Nature communications, 6, 7882. doi:10.1038/ncomms8882

21. Ye, D., Guan, K. L., & Xiong, Y. (2018). Metabolism, Activity, and Targeting of D- and L-2-Hydroxyglutarates. Trends in cancer, 4(2), 151–165. doi:10.1016/j.trecan.2017.12.005

CHAPTER 3

1. Holy Bible Modern English Version. (2014). Proverbs 16:18. Lake Mary, FL: Charisma House.

2. Holy Bible Modern English Version. (2014). 1 Samuel 17:50. Lake Mary, FL: Charisma House.

3. Tzu, S. (2012). The Art of War, 5-8. Minneapolis, MN: Filiquarian Publishing.

4. NCI Dictionary of Cancer Terms. (n.d.). Retrieved from https://www.cancer.gov/publications/dictionaries/cancer-terms

5. Morgan G, Ward R, Barton M. The contribution of cytotoxic chemotherapy to 5-year survival in adult malignancies. *Clin Oncol (R Coll Radiol)*. 2004;16(8):549-560. doi:10.1016/j.clon.2004.06.007

6. Staging. (n.d.). Retrieved from https://www.cancer.gov/about-cancer/diagnosis-staging/staging

7. Gilbert, R. (2014). Laughter therapy: promoting health and wellbeing. Nursing & Residential Care, 16(7), 392-395.

8. Exposure to chemical in Roundup increases risk for cancer, study finds. (2019, February 14). Retrieved from https://www.sciencedaily.com/releases/2019/02/190214093359.htm

9. Radon and Cancer. (n.d.). Retrieved from https://www.cancer.gov/about-cancer/causes-prevention/risk/substances/radon/radon-fact-sheet

10. LeBlanc, T. W., & Kamal, A. H. (2017, May 01). Assessing Psychological Toxicity and Patient-Reported Distress as the Sixth Vital Sign in Cancer Care and Clinical Trials. Retrieved from https://journalofethics.ama-assn.org/article/assessing-psychological-toxicity-and-patient-reported-distress-sixth-vital-sign-cancer-care-and/2017-05

CHAPTER 4

1. Storey, M., Jordan, S. An overview of the immune system. Nursing Standard [serial online]. December 17, 2008; 23(15-17):47-56 10p.

2. High-Dose Vitamin C (PDQ®)–Patient Version. Retrieved from https://www.cancer.gov/about-cancer/treatment/cam/patient/vitamin-c-pdq

3. Laetrile/Amygdalin (PDQ®)–Patient Version. Retrieved from https://www.cancer.gov/about-cancer/treatment/cam/patient/laetrile-pdq

4. Angiogenesis Inhibitors. (n.d.). Retrieved from https://www.cancer.gov/about-cancer/treatment/types/immunotherapy/angiogenesis-inhibitors-fact-sheet

5. Yang, S. P., Morita, I., & Murota, S. I. (1998, August). Eicosapentaenoic acid attenuates vascular endothelial growth factor-induced proliferation via inhibiting Flk-1 receptor expression in bovine carotid artery endothelial cells. Retrieved from https://www.ncbi.nlm.nih.gov/pubmed/9648921

6. Spencer, L., Mann, C., Metcalfe, M., Webb, M. B., Pollard, C., Spencer, D., ... Dennison, A. (2009, August). The effect of omega-3 FAs on tumour angiogenesis and their therapeutic potential. Retrieved from https://www.ncbi.nlm.nih.gov/pubmed/19493674

7. Bruns, H., Kazanavicius, D., Schultze, D., Saeedi, M. A., Yamanaka, K., Strupas, K., & Schemmer, P. (2016, November). Glycine inhibits angiogenesis in colorectal cancer: role of endothelial cells. Retrieved from https://www.ncbi.nlm.nih.gov/pubmed/27351202

8. Yamashina, S., Konno, A., Wheeler, M. D., Rusyn, I., Rusyn, E. V., Cox, A. D., & Thurman, R. G. (2001). Endothelial cells contain a glycine-gated chloride channel. Retrieved from https://www.ncbi.nlm.nih.gov/pubmed/11962256

9. McCarty, M. F., Iloki-Assanga, S., Lujan, L. M. L., & DiNicolantonio, J. J. (2019, February). Activated glycine receptors may decrease endosomal NADPH oxidase activity by opposing ClC-3-mediated efflux of chloride from endosomes. Retrieved from https://www.ncbi.nlm.nih.gov/pubmed/30696582

10. Shankar, S., Ganapathy, S., Hingorani, S. R., & Srivastava, R. K. (2008, January 1). EGCG inhibits growth, invasion, angiogenesis and metastasis of pancreatic cancer. Retrieved from https://www.ncbi.nlm.nih.gov/pubmed/17981559

11. Jung, Y. D., Kim, M. S., Shin, B. A., Chay, K. O., Ahn, B. W., Liu, W., ... Ellis, L. M. (2001, March 23). EGCG, a major component of green tea, inhibits tumour growth by inhibiting VEGF induction in human colon carcinoma cells. Retrieved from https://www.ncbi.nlm.nih.gov/pubmed/11259102

12. Jung, Y. D., & Ellis, L. M. (2001, December). Inhibition of tumour invasion and angiogenesis by epigallocatechin gallate (EGCG), a major component of green tea. Retrieved from https://www.ncbi.nlm.nih.gov/pubmed/11846837

13. Kondo, T., Ohta, T., Igura, K., Hara, Y., & Kaji, K. (2002, June 28). Tea catechins inhibit angiogenesis in vitro, measured by human endothelial cell growth, migration and tube formation, through inhibition of VEGF receptor binding. Retrieved from https://www.ncbi.nlm.nih.gov/pubmed/12175544

14. Zhu, B.-H., Zhan, W.-H., Li, Z.-R., Wang, Z., He, Y.-L., Peng, J.-S., ... Zhang, C.-H. (2007, February 28). (-)-Epigallocatechin-3-gallate inhibits growth of gastric cancer by reducing VEGF production and angiogenesis. Retrieved from https://www.ncbi.nlm.nih.gov/pubmed/17451194

15. Zhu, B.-H., Chen, H.-Y., Zhan, W.-H., Wang, C.-Y., Cai, S.-R., Wang, Z., ... He, Y.-L. (2011, May 14). (-)-Epigallocatechin-3-gallate inhibits VEGF expression induced by IL-6 via Stat3 in gastric cancer. Retrieved from https://www.ncbi.nlm.nih.gov/pubmed/21633597

16. Saini, M. K., & Sanyal, S. N. (2014, June). Targeting angiogenic pathway for chemoprevention of experimental colon cancer using C-phycocyanin as cyclooxygenase-2 inhibitor. Retrieved from https://www.ncbi.nlm.nih.gov/pubmed/24861078

17. Koníčková, R., Vaňková, K., Vaníková, J., Váňová, K., Muchová, L., Subhanová, I., ... Vítek, L. (2014). Anticancer effects of blue-green alga Spirulina platensis, a natural source of bilirubin-like tetrapyrrolic compounds. Retrieved from https://www.ncbi.nlm.nih.gov/pubmed/24552870

18. Kim, J. Y., & Kim, Y.M. (2019). Tumor endothelial cells as a potential target of metronomic chemotherapy. Retrieved from https://www.ncbi.nlm.nih.gov/pubmed/30604201

CHAPTER 5

1. History.com Editors. (2009, November 16). Muhammad Ali wins the Rumble in the Jungle. Retrieved from https://www.history.com/this-day-in-history/muhammad-ali-wins-the-rumble-in-the-jungle

2. Tzu, S. (2012). The Art of War. Minneapolis, MN: Filiquarian Publishing.

3. Center for Drug Evaluation and Research. (n.d.). Development & Approval Process (Drugs). Retrieved from https://www.fda.gov/drugs/development-approval-process-drugs

4. FOLFOX. (n.d.). Retrieved from https://www.cancer.gov/about-cancer/treatment/drugs/folfox

5. Wright, N., Xia, J., Cantuaria, G., Klimov, S., Jones, M., Neema, P., ... Aneja, R. (2017). Distinctions in Breast Tumor Recurrence Patterns Post-Therapy among Racially Distinct Populations. Plos One, 12(1), e0170095. https://doi.org/10.1371/journal.pone.0170095

6. Jang, J.-Y., Kang, J. S., Han, Y., Heo, J. S., Choi, S. H., Choi, D. W., ... Kim, S.-W. (2017). Long-term outcomes and recurrence patterns of standard versus extended pancreatectomy for pancreatic head cancer: a multicenter prospective randomized controlled study. Journal Of Hepato-Biliary-Pancreatic Sciences, 24(7), 426–433. https://doi.org/10.1002/jhbp.465

7. Ahmad, U., Hakim, A. H., Tang, A., Tong, M. Z., Bribriesco, A., Budev, M., ... Murthy, S. C. (2019). Patterns of Recurrence and Overall Survival in Incidental Lung Cancer in Explanted Lungs. The Annals of Thoracic Surgery, 107(3), 891–896. https://doi.org/10.1016/j.athoracsur.2018.09.022

CHAPTER 6

1. Waxman, O. B. (2016, June 3). Teenage Mutant Ninja Turtles: Origins and Real Ninja History. Retrieved from https://time.com/4351785/teenage-mutant-ninja-turtles-origins-history-out-shadows/.
2. Luquet, G. (2012). Biomineralizations: insights and prospects from crustaceans. Retrieved from https://www.ncbi.nlm.nih.gov/pmc/articles/PMC3335408/.
3. Maggini, S., Pierre, A., & Calder, P. C. (2018, October 17). Immune Function and Micronutrient Requirements Change over the Life Course. Retrieved from https://www.ncbi.nlm.nih.gov/pmc/articles/PMC6212925/.
4. Bates, S. E. (2012, January 1). On Drug Development, Chance, and the Prepared Mind. Retrieved from https://clincancerres.aacrjournals.org/content/18/1/22
5. "Research." MPI - Biology of ageing. Accessed November 16, 2019. https://www.age.mpg.de/science/research-laboratories/partridge/research/.
6. Weroha, S John, and Paul Haluska. "The Insulin-like Growth Factor System in Cancer." Endocrinology and metabolism clinics of North America. U.S. National Library of Medicine, June 2012. https://www.ncbi.nlm.nih.gov/pmc/articles/PMC3614012/.
7. Harvard Health Publishing. (n.d.). The lowdown on glycemic index and glycemic load. Retrieved from https://www.health.harvard.edu/diseases-and-conditions/the-lowdown-on-glycemic-index-and-glycemic-load.
8. NCI Dictionary of Cancer Terms. (n.d.). Retrieved from https://www.cancer.gov/publications/dictionaries/cancer-terms/def/glycemic-index.
9. McCarty, M.F. Insulin and IGF-I as determinants of low "Western" cancer rates in the rural third world. Int J Epidemiol 2004 August;33(4):908-10.
10. McCarty, M.F. Minimizing the cancer-promotional activity of COX-2 as a central strategy in cancer prevention. Med Hypotheses 2012 January;78(1):45-57.

11. Kwon, K.H. Barve, A. Yu, S. Huang, M.T. Kong, A.N. Cancer chemoprevention by phytochemicals: potential molecular targets, biomarkers and animal models. Acta Pharmacol Sin 2007 September;28(9):1409-21.

12. Fahey JW, Talalay P, Kensler TW. Notes from the field: "green" chemoprevention as frugal medicine. Cancer Prev Res (Phila) 2012 February;5(2):179-88.

13. Hallberg, L. Iron requirements and bioavailability of dietary iron. Experientia Suppl 1983;44:223-44.

14. Luo Y, Han Z, Chin SM, Linn S. Three chemically distinct types of oxidants formed by iron-mediated Fenton reactions in the presence of DNA. Proc Natl Acad Sci U S A 1994 December 20;91(26):12438-42.

15. Nakano M, Kawanishi Y, Kamohara S et al. Oxidative DNA damage (8-hydroxydeoxyguanosine) and body iron status: a study on 2507 healthy people. Free Radic Biol Med 2003 October 1;35(7):826-32.

16. Alexander D, Ball MJ, Mann J. Nutrient intake and haematological status of vegetarians and age-sex matched omnivores. Eur J Clin Nutr 1994 August;48(8):538-46.

17. Overvik E, Kleman M, Berg I, Gustafsson JA. Influence of creatine, amino acids and water on the formation of the mutagenic heterocyclic amines found in cooked meat. Carcinogenesis 1989 December;10(12):2293-301.

18. Skog KI, Johansson MA, Jagerstad MI. Carcinogenic heterocyclic amines in model systems and cooked foods: a review on formation, occurrence and intake. Food Chem Toxicol 1998 September;36(9-10):879-96.

19. Baserga R, Peruzzi F, Reiss K. The IGF-1 receptor in cancer biology. Int J Cancer 2003 December 20;107(6):873-7.

20. Moschos SJ, Mantzoros CS. The role of the IGF system in cancer: from basic to clinical studies and clinical applications. Oncology 2002;63(4):317-32.

21. Giovannucci E. Nutrition, insulin, insulin-like growth factors and cancer. Horm Metab Res 2003 November;35(11-12):694-704.

22. Pollak MN. Insulin-like growth factors and neoplasia. Novartis Found Symp 2004;262:84-98.

23. Yakar S, Pennisi P, Zhao H, Zhang Y, LeRoith D. Circulating IGF-1 and its role in cancer: lessons from the IGF-1 gene deletion (LID) mouse. Novartis Found Symp 2004;262:3-9.

24. Dunn SE, Kari FW, French J et al. Dietary restriction reduces insulin-like growth factor I levels, which modulates apoptosis, cell proliferation, and tumor progression in p53-deficient mice. Cancer Res 1997 November 1;57(21):4667-72.

25. Allen NE, Appleby PN, Davey GK, Key TJ. Hormones and diet: low insulin-like growth factor-I but normal bioavailable androgens in vegan men. Br J Cancer 2000 July;83(1):95-7.

26. Allen NE, Appleby PN, Davey GK, Kaaks R, Rinaldi S, Key TJ. The associations of diet with serum insulin-like growth factor I and its main binding proteins in 292 women meat-eaters, vegetarians, and vegans. Cancer Epidemiol Biomarkers Prev 2002 November;11(11):1441-8.

27. Fontana L, Klein S, Holloszy JO. Long-term low-protein, low-calorie diet and endurance exercise modulate metabolic factors associated with cancer risk. Am J Clin Nutr 2006 December;84(6):1456-62.

28. Fontana L, Weiss EP, Villareal DT, Klein S, Holloszy JO. Long-term effects of calorie or protein restriction on serum IGF-1 and IGFBP-3 concentration in humans. Aging Cell 2008 October;7(5):681-7.

29. Fontana L, Adelaiye RM, Rastelli AL et al. Dietary protein restriction inhibits tumor growth in human xenograft models. Oncotarget 2013 December;4(12):2451-61.

30. Ngo TH, Barnard RJ, Tymchuk CN, Cohen P, Aronson WJ. Effect of diet and exercise on serum insulin, IGF-I, and IGFBP-1 levels and growth of LNCaP cells in vitro (United States). Cancer Causes Control 2002 December;13(10):929-35.

31. Ngo TH, Barnard RJ, Leung PS, Cohen P, Aronson WJ. Insulin-like growth factor I (IGF-I) and IGF binding protein-1 modulate prostate cancer cell growth and apoptosis: possible mediators for the effects of diet and exercise on cancer cell survival. Endocrinology 2003 June;144(6):2319-24.

32. Ornish D, Weidner G, Fair WR et al. Intensive lifestyle changes may affect the progression of prostate cancer. J Urol 2005 September;174(3):1065-9.

33. Frattaroli J, Weidner G, Dnistrian AM et al. Clinical events in prostate cancer lifestyle trial: results from two years of follow-up. Urology 2008 December;72(6):1319-23.

34. Satillaro AJ. Recalled by life. New York City: Avon Books; 1982.

35. McCarty MF. GCN2 and FGF21 are likely mediators of the protection from cancer, autoimmunity, obesity, and diabetes afforded by vegan diets. Med Hypotheses 2014 September;83(3):365-71.

36. Gallinetti J, Harputlugil E, Mitchell JR. Amino acid sensing in dietary-restriction-mediated longevity: roles of signal-transducing kinases GCN2 and TOR. Biochem J 2013 January 1;449(1):1-10.

37. Zhang Y, Xie Y, Berglund ED et al. The starvation hormone, fibroblast growth factor-21, extends lifespan in mice. Elife 2012;1:e00065.

38. Mendelsohn AR, Larrick JW. Fibroblast growth factor-21 is a promising dietary restriction mimetic. Rejuvenation Res 2012 December;15(6):624-8.

39. Perrier S, Jarde T. Adiponectin, an anti-carcinogenic hormone? A systematic review on breast, colorectal, liver and prostate cancer. Curr Med Chem 2012;19(32):5501-12.

40. Adams AC, Kharitonenkov A. FGF21 drives a shift in adipokine tone to restore metabolic health. Aging (Albany NY) 2013 June;5(6):386-7.

41. McCarty MF, Barroso-Aranda J, Contreras F. The low-methionine content of vegan diets may make methionine restriction feasible as a life extension strategy. Med Hypotheses 2009 February;72(2):125-8.

42. Campbell TC, Campbell TM. The China study : The most comprehensive study of nutrition ever conducted and the startling Implications for diet, weight Loss and long-term health. Benbella Books; 2006.

43. NCI Dictionary of Cancer Terms. (n.d.). Retrieved from https://www.cancer.gov/publications/dictionaries/cancer-terms/def/cachexia.

44. Todorov, P. T., Field, W. N., & Tisdale, M. J. (1999, August). Role of a proteolysis-inducing factor (PIF) in cachexia induced by a human melanoma (G361). Retrieved from https://www.ncbi.nlm.nih.gov/pmc/articles/PMC2374268/.

45. Giacosa, A., & Rondanelli, M. (2008, April). Fish oil and treatment of cancer cachexia. Retrieved from https://www.ncbi.nlm.nih.gov/pmc/articles/PMC2311497/.

46. Gullett, N. P., Mazurak, V. C., Hebbar, G., & Ziegler, T. R. (2011). Nutritional interventions for cancer-induced cachexia. Retrieved from https://www.ncbi.nlm.nih.gov/pmc/articles/PMC3106221/.

CHAPTER 7

1. Throw shade. (n.d.). Retrieved from https://www.urbandictionary.com/define.php?term=Throw shade.

2. Chen, L., Deng, H., Cui, H., Fang, J., Zuo, Z., Deng, J., ... Zhao, L. (2017, December 14). Inflammatory responses and inflammation-associated diseases in organs. Retrieved from https://www.ncbi.nlm.nih.gov/pmc/articles/PMC5805548/.

3. Gerondakis, S., & Siebenlist, U. (2010, May). Roles of the NF-kappaB pathway in lymphocyte development and function. Retrieved from https://www.ncbi.nlm.nih.gov/pmc/articles/PMC2857169/.

4. Xia, Y., Shen, S., & Verma, I. M. (2014, September). NF-κB, an active player in human cancers. Retrieved from https://www.ncbi.nlm.nih.gov/pmc/articles/PMC4155602/.

5. Park, M. H., & Hong, J. T. (2016, March 29). Roles of NF-κB in Cancer and Inflammatory Diseases and Their Therapeutic Approaches. Retrieved from https://www.ncbi.nlm.nih.gov/pmc/articles/PMC4931664/.

6. Taniguchi, K., & Karin, M. (2018, January 22). NF-κB, inflammation, immunity and cancer: coming of age. Retrieved from https://www.nature.com/articles/nri.2017.142.

7. Aggarwal, B. B., & Sung, B. (2011, November 1). NF-κB in Cancer: A Matter of Life and Death. Retrieved from https://cancerdiscovery.aacrjournals.org/content/1/6/469.

8. Xu, L., Botchway, B. O. A., Zhang, S., Zhou, J., & Liu, X. (2018, October 4). Inhibition of NF-κB Signaling Pathway by Resveratrol Improves Spinal Cord Injury. Retrieved from https://www.ncbi.nlm.nih.gov/pmc/articles/PMC6180204/.

9. Zarghi, A., & Arfaei, S. (2011). Selective COX-2 Inhibitors: A Review of Their Structure-Activity Relationships. Retrieved from https://www.ncbi.nlm.nih.gov/pmc/articles/PMC3813081/.

10. Elwood, P. C., Morgan, G., Pickering, J. E., Galante, J., Weightman, A. L., Morris, D., ... Dolwani, S. (2016, April 20). Aspirin in the Treatment of Cancer: Reductions in Metastatic Spread and in Mortality: A Systematic Review and Meta-Analyses of Published Studies. Retrieved from https://www.ncbi.nlm.nih.gov/pmc/articles/PMC4838306/.

11. Aspirin to Reduce Cancer Risk. (n.d.). Retrieved from https://www.cancer.gov/about-cancer/causes-prevention/research/aspirin-cancer-risk.

12. Portnow, J., Suleman, S., Grossman, S. A., Eller, S., & Carson, K. (2002, January). A cyclooxygenase-2 (COX-2) inhibitor compared with dexamethasone in a survival study of rats with intracerebral 9L gliosarcomas. Retrieved from https://www.ncbi.nlm.nih.gov/pubmed/11772429.

13. Vučković, S., Srebro, D., Vujović, K. S., Vučetić, Č., & Prostran, M. (2018, November 13). Cannabinoids and Pain: New Insights From Old Molecules. Retrieved from https://www.ncbi.nlm.nih.gov/pmc/articles/PMC6277878/.

14. Wang, J., Wang, Y., Tong, M., Pan, H., & Li, D. (2019, January 1). New Prospect for Cancer Cachexia: Medical Cannabinoid. Retrieved from https://www.ncbi.nlm.nih.gov/pmc/articles/PMC6360413/.

15. Griffiths, J. R. (1991, September). Are cancer cells acidic? Retrieved from https://www.ncbi.nlm.nih.gov/pmc/articles/PMC1977628/.

16. Donaldson, A. E., & Lamont, I. L. (2013, November 21). Biochemistry changes that occur after death: potential markers for determining post-mortem interval. Retrieved from https://www.ncbi.nlm.nih.gov/pmc/articles/PMC3836773/.

17. Reddy, A., Norris, D. F., Momeni, S. S., Waldo, B., & Ruby, J. D. (2016, April). The pH of beverages in the United States. Retrieved from https://www.ncbi.nlm.nih.gov/pmc/articles/PMC4808596/.

18. Faes, S., & Dormond, O. (2015, December 30). Systemic Buffers in Cancer Therapy: The Example of Sodium Bicarbonate; Stupid Idea or Wise Remedy? Retrieved from https://www.omicsonline.org/open-access/systemic-buffers-in-cancer-therapy-the-example-of-sodium-bicarbonatestupid-idea-or-wise-remedy-2161-0444-1000314.php?aid=65744.

19. Zhang, H. (2017, March). Will cancer cells be defeated by sodium bicarbonate? Retrieved from https://www.ncbi.nlm.nih.gov/pmc/articles/PMC5954837/.

20. Robey, I. F., & Nesbit, L. A. (2013). Investigating mechanisms of alkalinization for reducing primary breast tumor invasion. Retrieved from https://www.ncbi.nlm.nih.gov/pmc/articles/PMC3722989/.

21. Robey, I. F., Baggett, B. K., Kirkpatrick, N. D., Roe, D. J., Dosescu, J., Sloane, B. F., ... Gillies, R. J. (2009, March 15). Bicarbonate increases tumor pH and inhibits spontaneous metastases. Retrieved from https://www.ncbi.nlm.nih.gov/pmc/articles/PMC2834485/

22. Markovic, M. (2007, December 21). Short Term Hyperthermia Prevents Activation of Proinflammatory Genes in Type B Synoviocytes by Blocking the Activation of the Transcription Factor NF-κB. Retrieved from https://www.ncbi.nlm.nih.gov/pmc/articles/PMC5869223/.

CHAPTER 8

1. Homer. (1999). The Iliad: with an English translation by A.T. Murray. London: Harvard University Press.

2. History.com Editors. (2011, March 21). Achilles. Retrieved from https://www.history.com/topics/ancient-history/achilles.

3. Tzu, S. (2012). The Art of War. Minneapolis, MN: Filiquarian Publishing.

4. Housman, G., Byler, S., Heerboth, S., Lapinska, K., Longacre, M., Snyder, N., & Sarkar, S. (2014, September 5). Drug resistance in cancer: an overview. Retrieved from https://www.ncbi.nlm.nih.gov/pmc/articles/PMC4190567/.

5. Goldstein, D. S. (2010, November). Adrenal responses to stress. Retrieved from https://www.ncbi.nlm.nih.gov/pmc/articles/PMC3056281/.

6. Segerstrom, S. C., & Miller, G. E. (2004, July). Psychological stress and the human immune system: a meta-analytic study of 30 years of inquiry. Retrieved from https://www.ncbi.nlm.nih.gov/pmc/articles/PMC1361287/.

7. Hannibal, K. E., & Bishop, M. D. (2014, December). Chronic stress, cortisol dysfunction, and pain: a psychoneuroendocrine rationale for stress management in pain rehabilitation. Retrieved from https://www.ncbi.nlm.nih.gov/pmc/articles/PMC4263906/.

8. Perkins, A., & Liu, G. (2016, February 1). Primary Brain Tumors in Adults: Diagnosis and Treatment. Retrieved from https://www.aafp.org/afp/2016/0201/p211.html.

CHAPTER 9

1. Clavo, B., Rodríguez-Esparragón, F., Rodríguez-Abreu, D., Martínez-Sánchez, G., Llontop, P., Aguiar-Bujanda, D., ... Santana-Rodríguez, N. (2019, November 26). Modulation of Oxidative Stress by Ozone Therapy in the Prevention and Treatment of Chemotherapy-Induced Toxicity: Review and Prospects. Retrieved from https://www.ncbi.nlm.nih.gov/pmc/articles/PMC6943601/

2. Integrative, P. D. Q., Alternative, & Board, and C. T. E. (2019, October 25). Laetrile/Amygdalin (PDQ®). Retrieved from https://www.ncbi.nlm.nih.gov/books/NBK65988/

3. Shi, J., Chen, Q., Xu, M., Xia, Q., Zheng, T., Teng, J., ... Fan, L. (2019, June). Recent updates and future perspectives about amygdalin as a potential anticancer agent: A review. Retrieved from https://www.ncbi.nlm.nih.gov/pmc/articles/PMC6558459/

4. Laetrile/Amygdalin (PDQ®)–Patient Version. (n.d.). Retrieved from https://www.cancer.gov/about-cancer/treatment/cam/patient/laetrile-pdq.

5. National Cancer Institute. Laetrile/Amygdalin (PDQ®) Overview. http://www.cancer.gov/about-cancer/treatment/cam/patient/laetrile-pdq#section/_3

6. Zuoqing S, Xiaohong X. Advanced research on anti-tumor effects of amygdalin. Journal of Cancer Research & Therapeutics [serial online]. Aug2014 Special Issue 2014;10(S5):C3-C7.

7. Cancer Research UK. How Cancer Grows. http://www.cancerresearchuk.org/about-cancer/what-is-cancer/how-cancers-grow

8. Mirmiranpour H, Khaghani S, Esteghamati A, et al. Amygdalin inhibits angiogenesis in the cultured endothelial cells of diabetic rats. Indian Journal of Pathology & Microbiology [serial online]. April 2012;55(2):211-214.

9. ChenY,MaJ,LiF,etal. Amygdalin induces apoptosis in human cervical cancer cell line HeLa cells. Immunopharmacology and Immunotoxicology [serial online]. February 2013;35(1):43-51.

10. Makarević J, Rutz J, Blaheta R, et al. Amygdalin Influences Bladder Cancer Cell Adhesion and Invasion In Vitro. PlosONE [serial online]. October 2014;9(10):1-11.

11. Paoletti I, De Gregorio V, Baroni A, Tufano M, Donnarumma G, Perez J. Amygdalin analogues inhibit IFN-γ signalling and reduce the inflammatory response in human epidermal keratinocytes. Inflammation [serial online]. December 2013;36(6):1316-1326.

12. Yang H, Chang H, Kim C, et al. Amygdalin suppresses lipopolysaccharide-induced expressions of cyclooxygenase-2 and inducible nitric oxide synthase in mouse BV2 microglial cells. Neurological Research [serial online]. 2007;29 Suppl 1:S59-S64.

13. Zhu H, Chang L, Li W, Liu H. Effect of amygdalin on the proliferation of hyperoxia-exposed type II alveolar epithelial cells isolated from premature rat. Journal Of Huazhong University of Science and Technology. Medical Sciences = Hua Zhong Ke Ji Da Xue Xue Bao. Yi Xue Ying De Wen Ban = Huazhong Keji Daxue Xuebao. Yixue Yingdewen Ban [serial online]. 2004;24(3):223-225.

14. National Cancer Act of 1971. (n.d.). Retrieved from https://www.cancer.gov/about-nci/overview/history/national-cancer-act-1971

15. Elflein, J. (2019, November 6). Deaths by cancer U.S. 1950-2017. Retrieved from https://www.statista.com/statistics/184566/deaths-by-cancer-in-the-us-since-1950/

16. American Cancer Society. (2019) Cancer Facts & Figures 2019. Atlanta: American Cancer Society.

17. Facts & Figures 2018: Rate of Deaths From Cancer Continues Decline. (n.d.). Retrieved from https://www.cancer.org/latest-news/facts-and-figures-2018-rate-of-deaths-from-cancer-continues-decline.html

18. Prasad, V., & Mailankody, S. (2017, November 1). Research and Development Spending to Bring a Single Cancer Drug to Market and Revenues After Approval. Retrieved from https://www.ncbi.nlm.nih.gov/pmc/articles/PMC5710275/

19. Dolgin, E. (2018, March 7). Bringing down the cost of cancer treatment. Retrieved from https://www.nature.com/articles/d41586-018-02483-3

20. Medicare. (2020). Your Medicare Benefits. Retrieved from https://www.medicare.gov/Pubs/pdf/10116-Your-Medicare-Benefits.pdf

21. General cancer information. (2019, September 27). Retrieved from https://www.cancerresearchuk.org/about-cancer/cancer-in-general/treatment/access-to-treatment/private-nhs

22. Integrative, P. D. Q., Alternative, & Board, and C. T. E. (2013, February 8). High-Dose Vitamin C (PDQ®). Retrieved from https://www.ncbi.nlm.nih.gov/books/NBK121338/

23. Jacobs, C., Hutton, B., Ng, T., Shorr, R., & Clemons, M. (2015, February). Is there a role for oral or intravenous ascorbate (Vitamin C) in treating patients with cancer? A systematic review. Retrieved from https://www.ncbi.nlm.nih.gov/pubmed/25601965

24. J., E., Dachs, U., G., & Campbell. (2014, September 29). Current Limitations of Murine Models in Oncology for Ascorbate Research. Retrieved from https://www.frontiersin.org/articles/10.3389/fonc.2014.00282/full

25. Padayatty, S. J., Riordan, H. D., Hewitt, S. M., Katz, A., Hoffer, L. J., & Levine, M. (2006, March 28). Intravenously administered Vitamin C as cancer therapy: three cases. Retrieved from https://www.ncbi.nlm.nih.gov/pmc/articles/PMC1405876/

26. High Dose IV Vitamin C and Metastatic Breast Cancer: A Case Report. (2019, January 16). Retrieved from https://isom.ca/article/high-dose-iv-vitamin-c-metastatic-breast-cancer-case-report/

27. Seo, M.-S., Kim, J.-K., & Shim, J.-Y. (2015, September). High-Dose Vitamin C Promotes Regression of Multiple Pulmonary Metastases Originating from Hepatocellular Carcinoma. Retrieved from https://www.ncbi.nlm.nih.gov/pmc/articles/PMC4541681/

28. Jackson, J., Riordan, H., Bramhall, N., Neathery, S. (2002). Sixteen-Year History with High Dose Vitamin C Treatment For Various Types of Cancer and Other Diseases. Journal of Orthomolecular Cancer. Vol. 17 (2).

29. Mandal, A. (2019, May 3). What is Oxidative Stress? Retrieved from https://www.news-medical.net/health/What-is-Oxidative-Stress.aspx

30. Elzbieta, Szczepanska, Joanna, Blasiak, & Janusz. (2019, December 24). Pro- and Antioxidant Effects of Vitamin C in Cancer in correspondence to Its Dietary and Pharmacological Concentrations. Retrieved from https://www.hindawi.com/journals/omcl/2019/7286737/

31. Oberley, T. D., & Oberley, L. W. (1997, April). Antioxidant enzyme levels in cancer. Retrieved from https://www.ncbi.nlm.nih.gov/pubmed/9151141

32. Why high-dose Vitamin C kills cancer cells. (2017, January 9). Retrieved from https://www.sciencedaily.com/releases/2017/01/170109134014.htm

33. Traub, M., Traub, M., Anderson, P., & AuthorsMichael Traub. (n.d.). Intravenous Vitamin C in Cancer. Retrieved from https://www.naturalmedicinejournal.com/journal/2014-02/intravenous-vitamin-c-cancer

34. Kato, Y., Ozawa, S., Miyamoto, C., Maehata, Y., Suzuki, A., Maeda, T., & Baba, Y. (2013, September 3). Acidic extracellular microenvironment and cancer. Retrieved from https://www.ncbi.nlm.nih.gov/pmc/articles/PMC3849184/

35. van Gorkom, G. N. Y., Lookermans, E. L., Van Elssen, C. H. M. J., & Bos, G. M. J. (2019, April 28). The Effect of Vitamin C (Ascorbic Acid) in the Treatment of Patients with Cancer: A Systematic Review. Retrieved from https://www.ncbi.nlm.nih.gov/pmc/articles/PMC6566697/

36. Increasing the Effectiveness of Intravenous Vitamin C as an Anticancer Agent. (2017, March 1). Retrieved from https://isom.ca/article/increasing-the-effectiveness-of-intravenous-vitamin-c-as-an-anticancer-agent/

37. Van Gorkom, G. N. Y., Lookermans, E. L., Van Elssen, C. H. M. J., & Bos, G. M. J. (2019, April 28). The Effect of Vitamin C (Ascorbic Acid) in the Treatment of Patients with Cancer: A Systematic Review. Retrieved from https://www.ncbi.nlm.nih.gov/pmc/articles/PMC6566697/

38. Nauman, G., Gray, J. C., Parkinson, R., Levine, M., & Paller, C. J. (2018, July 12). Systematic Review of Intravenous Ascorbate in Cancer Clinical Trials. Retrieved from https://www.ncbi.nlm.nih.gov/pmc/articles/PMC6071214/

39. Mikirova, N., Casciari, J., Rogers, A. et al. Effect of high-dose intravenous Vitamin C on inflammation in cancer patients. J Transl Med 10, 189 (2012). https://doi.org/10.1186/1479-5876-10-189

40. Elzbieta, Szczepanska, Joanna, Blasiak, & Janusz. (2019, December 24). Pro- and Antioxidant Effects of Vitamin C in Cancer in correspondence to Its Dietary and Pharmacological Concentrations. Retrieved from https://www.hindawi.com/journals/omcl/2019/7286737/

41. Klimant, E., Wright, H., Rubin, D., Seely, D., & Markman, M. (2018, April). Intravenous Vitamin C in the supportive care of cancer patients: a review and rational approach. Retrieved from https://www.ncbi.nlm.nih.gov/pmc/articles/PMC5927785/

CHAPTER 10

1. Q&A: Ryan on the art of the strikeout. (2016, September 10). Retrieved from https://www.mlb.com/news/nolan-ryan-tells-how-to-strike-out-a-batter-c200539502.

2. FIPmyWHIP. (2017, June 10). Nolan Ryan's incredible career should earn him the title of "best pitcher ever". Retrieved from https://www.beyondtheboxscore.com/2017/6/10/15759862/nolan-ryan-rangers-astros-angels-mets-strikeouts-velocity-record-blisters-the-best-pitcher-ever.

3. Wire, S. I. (2015, April 22). Pitching by numbers: 'Fastball' provides scientific looks at baseball. Retrieved from https://www.si.com/extra-mustard/2015/04/22/fastball-pitching-documentary-mlb.

4. Bobby Grich Stats. (n.d.). Retrieved from https://www.baseball-reference.com/players/g/grichbo01.shtml.

5. Coffey, A. (n.d.). Nolan Ryan tosses his fourth no-hitter. Retrieved from https://baseballhall.org/discover-more/stories/inside-pitch/nolan-ryan-tosses-his-fourth-no-hitter

6. 2010, The Ultimate Quotable Einstein, Edited by Alice Calaprice, Section: Misattributed to Einstein, Quote Page 474, Princeton University Press, Princeton, New Jersey.

7. Oxford Electronic Dictionary. (n.d.). Retrieved from https://www.oed.com/.

8. National Cancer Institute (NCI). (2017, October 18). Retrieved from https://www.nih.gov/about-nih/what-we-do/nih-almanac/national-cancer-institute-nci.

9. Cancer Survivorship --- United States, 1971--2001. (n.d.). Retrieved from https://www.cdc.gov/mmwr/preview/mmwrhtml/mm5324a3.htm

10. Silverberg, E., & Holleb, A. I. (2008, December 30). Cancer statistics 1973. Retrieved from https://onlinelibrary.wiley.com/doi/pdf/10.3322/canjclin.23.1.2.

11. Cancer of Any Site - Cancer Stat Facts. (n.d.). Retrieved from https://seer.cancer.gov/statfacts/html/all.html.

12. Gianfaldoni, S., Gianfaldoni, R., Wollina, U., Lotti, J., Tchernev, G., & Lotti, T. (2017, July 18). An Overview on Radiotherapy: From Its History to Its Current Applications in Dermatology. Retrieved from https://www.ncbi.nlm.nih.gov/pmc/articles/PMC5535674/.

13. Tian, X., Liu, K., Hou, Y., Cheng, J., & Zhang, J. (2018, January). The evolution of proton beam therapy: Current and future status. Retrieved from https://www.ncbi.nlm.nih.gov/pmc/articles/PMC5772792/.

14. Shields, R. K., & Dudley-Javoroski, S. (2003, March). Musculoskeletal deterioration and hemicorporectomy after spinal cord injury. Retrieved from https://www.ncbi.nlm.nih.gov/pmc/articles/PMC4042312/.

15. Janis, J. E., Ahmad, J., Lemmon, J. A., Barnett, C. C., Morrill, K. C., & McClelland, R. N. (2009, October). A 25-year experience with hemicorporectomy for terminal pelvic osteomyelitis. Retrieved from https://www.ncbi.nlm.nih.gov/pubmed/19935300.

16. Janis, J. E., Ahmad, J., Lemmon, J. A., Barnett, C. C., Morrill, K. C., & McClelland, R. N. (2009, October). A 25-year experience with hemicorporectomy for terminal pelvic osteomyelitis. Retrieved from https://www.ncbi.nlm.nih.gov/pubmed/19935300.

17. Marks, L. B. (2019). Mastectomy May Be an Inferior Oncologic Approach Compared to Breast Preservation. International Journal of Radiation Oncology • Biology • Physics, Volume 103(1):78-80.

18. Holy Bible Modern English Version. (2014). Luke 6:31. Lake Mary, FL: Charisma House.

19. Holy Bible Modern English Version. (2014). Matthew 22:39. Lake Mary, FL: Charisma House.

20. COGBILL, C. L. (1965). Commando Procedures For Mouth Cancer. Arch Surg. 1965;90(1):153–156. doi:https://doi.org/10.1001/archsurg.1965.01320070155032

21. Kowalski, L. P., Hashimoto, I., & Magrin, J. (1993, October). End results of 114 extended "commando" operations for retromolar trigone carcinoma. Retrieved from https://www.ncbi.nlm.nih.gov/pubmed/8214296.

22. DeVita, V. T., & Chu, E. (2008, November 1). A History of Cancer Chemotherapy. Retrieved from https://cancerres.aacrjournals.org/content/68/21/864.

23. Morgan, G., Ward, R., & Barton, M. (2004, December). The contribution of cytotoxic chemotherapy to 5-year survival in adult malignancies. Retrieved from https://www.ncbi.nlm.nih.gov/pubmed/15630849.

24. Rizzieri, D. A., Johnson, J. L., Byrd, J. C., Lozanski, G., Blum, K. A., Powell, B. L., ... Alliance for Clinical Trials In Oncology (ACTION). (2014, April). Improved efficacy using rituximab and brief duration, high intensity chemotherapy with filgrastim support for Burkitt or aggressive lymphomas: cancer and Leukemia Group B study 10 002. Retrieved from https://www.ncbi.nlm.nih.gov/pmc/articles/PMC3996561/.

25. Ferioli, M., Zauli, G., Martelli, A. M., Vitale, M., McCubrey, J. A., Ultimo, S., ... Neri, L. M. (2018, February 8). Impact of physical exercise in cancer survivors during and after antineoplastic treatments. Retrieved from https://www.ncbi.nlm.nih.gov/pmc/articles/PMC5862633/.

26. Munzone, E., & Colleoni, M. (2015, November). Clinical overview of metronomic chemotherapy in breast cancer. Retrieved from https://www.ncbi.nlm.nih.gov/pubmed/26241939.

27. Hanahan, D., Bergers, G., & Bergsland, E. (2000, April 15). Less is more, regularly: metronomic dosing of cytotoxic drugs can target tumor angiogenesis in mice. Retrieved from https://www.jci.org/articles/view/9872.

28. Wu, K.-M. (2009, October 14). A New Classification of Prodrugs: Regulatory Perspectives. Retrieved from https://www.ncbi.nlm.nih.gov/pmc/articles/PMC3978533/.

29. Hennessy, Gauthier, Michaud, B., L., Hortobagyi, & Valero. (2005, May 12). Lower dose capecitabine has a more favorable therapeutic index in metastatic breast cancer: retrospective analysis of patients treated at M. D. Anderson Cancer Center and a review of capecitabine toxicity in the literature. Retrieved from https://academic.oup.com/annonc/article/16/8/1289/137346.

CHAPTER 11

1. Langley, N., Ryerson, F., & Woolf, E. A. (1939). The Wizard of Oz. Retrieved from https://sfy.ru/script/wizard_of_oz_1939.

2. Holy Bible Modern English Version. (2014). Psalm 23:4. Lake Mary, FL: Charisma House.

3. Tzu, S. (2012). The Art of War. Minneapolis, MN: Filiquarian Publishing.

4. Thompson, A. E. (2015, April 28). The Immune System. Retrieved from https://jamanetwork.com/journals/jama/fullarticle/2279715

5. Balloux, F., & van Dorp, L. (2017, October 19). Q&A: What are pathogens, and what have they done to and for us? Retrieved from https://www.ncbi.nlm.nih.gov/pmc/articles/PMC5648414/

6. NCI Dictionary of Cancer Terms. (n.d.). Retrieved from https://www.cancer.gov/publications/dictionaries/cancer-terms/search?contains=false&q=lymphocyte

7. NCI Dictionary of Cancer Terms. (n.d.). Retrieved from https://www.cancer.gov/publications/dictionaries/cancer-terms/def/nk-cell

8. NCI Dictionary of Cancer Terms. (n.d.). Retrieved from https://www.cancer.gov/publications/dictionaries/cancer-terms/def/t-reg

9. Wegiel, Barbara, Vuerich, Marta, Saeed, Seth, & Pankaj. (2018, July 9). Metabolic Switch in the Tumor Microenvironment Determines Immune Responses to Anticancer Therapy. Retrieved from https://www.frontiersin.org/articles/10.3389/fonc.2018.00284/full

10. Khan, F., Datta, S. D., Quddus, A., Vertefeuille, J. F., Burns, C. C., Jorba, J., & Wassilak, S. G. F. (2018, May 11). Progress Toward Polio Eradication - Worldwide, January 2016-March 2018. Retrieved from https://www.ncbi.nlm.nih.gov/pmc/articles/PMC5944975/

11. Vaccine. (n.d.). Retrieved from https://www.dictionary.com/browse/vaccine

12. Basu, P., Banerjee, D., Singh, P., Bhattacharya, C., & Biswas, J. (2013, October). Efficacy and safety of human papillomavirus vaccine for primary prevention of cervical cancer: A review of evidence from phase III trials and national programs. Retrieved from https://www.ncbi.nlm.nih.gov/pmc/articles/PMC3889021/

13. Tagliamonte, M., Petrizzo, A., Mauriello, A., Tornesello, M. L., Buonaguro, F. M., & Buonaguro, L. (2018, July 23). Potentiating cancer vaccine efficacy in liver cancer. Retrieved from https://www.ncbi.nlm.nih.gov/pmc/articles/PMC6169594/

14. NCI Dictionary of Cancer Terms. (n.d.). Retrieved from https://www.cancer.gov/publications/dictionaries/cancer-terms/search?contains=false&q=vaccine

15. Koski G, Cohen P, Roses R, Shuwen X, Czerniecki B. Reengineering dendritic cell-based anticancer vaccines. Immunological Reviews [serial online]. April 2008;222(1):256-276.

16. Hovden A, Appel S. The first dendritic cell-based therapeutic cancer vaccine is approved by the FDA. Scandinavian Journal of Immunology [serial online]. December 2010;72(6):554.

17. Definition of Dendritic Cell Vaccine - NCI Dictionary of Cancer Terms. National Cancer Institute. N.p., n.d. Web. 03 Nov. 2015.

18. Benencia F, Sprague L, McGinty J, Pate M, Muccioli M. Dendritic Cells the Tumor Microenvironment and the Challenges for an Effective Antitumor Vaccination. Journal of Biomedicine & Biotechnology [serial online]. January 2012;2012:1-15 15p.

19. Definition of Antigen-presenting Cell Vaccine - NCI Dictionary of Cancer Terms. National Cancer Institute. N.p., n.d. Web. 03 Nov. 2015.

20. Definition of Antigen - NCI Dictionary of Cancer Terms." National Cancer Institute. N.p., n.d. Web. 03 Nov. 2015.

21. Fleisher M. Criteria for tumor marker evaluation and utilization. (Cover story). MLO: Medical Laboratory Observer [serial online]. April 2003;35(4):16.

22. Mantia-Smaldone G, Chu C. A Review of Dendritic Cell Therapy for Cancer: Progress and Challenges. Biodrugs [serial online]. October 2013;27(5):453-468. Available from: Academic Search Complete, Ipswich, MA.

23. Koido S, Homma S, Tajiri H, et al. Immunologic monitoring of cellular responses by dendritic/tumor cell fusion vaccines. Journal Of Biomedicine & Biotechnology [serial online]. January 2011;:910836-910836 1p.

24. Karachaliou N, Gonzalez Cao M, Rosell R, et al. Understanding the function and dysfunction of the immune system in lung cancer: the role of immune checkpoints. Cancer Biology & Medicine [serial online]. June 2015;12(2):79-86.

25. Frank M, Kaufman J, Parveen S, Blachère N, Orange D, Darnell R. Dendritic cell vaccines containing lymphocytes produce improved immunogenicity in patients with cancer. Journal Of Translational Medicine [serial online]. December 15, 2014;12(1):199-219.

26. Anguille S, Van Acker H, Lion E, et al. Interleukin-15 Dendritic Cells Harness NK Cell Cytotoxic Effector Function in a Contact- and IL-15-Dependent Manner. Plos ONE [serial online]. May 2015;10(5):1-18.

27. Pampena M, Levy E, Zwirner N, Ferlazzo G. Natural killer cells as helper cells in dendritic cell cancer vaccines. Frontiers In Immunology [serial online]. January 2015;5:1-8.

28. Butterfield L. Dendritic cells in cancer immunotherapy clinical trials: are we making progress?. Frontiers In Immunology [serial online]. November 2013;4:1-22.

29. Human Tumor Antigens and Cancer Immunotherapy. Biomed Research International [serial online]. June 16, 2015;2015:1-17 17p.

30. Morel, P. A., & Turner, M. S. (2010). Designing the optimal vaccine: the importance of cytokines and dendritic cells. Retrieved from https://www.ncbi.nlm.nih.gov/pmc/articles/PMC3149857/

31. Fewkes, N. M., & Mackall, C. L. (2020). Novel gamma-chain cytokines as candidate immune modulators in immune therapies for cancer. Retrieved from https://www.ncbi.nlm.nih.gov/pmc/articles/PMC6959548/

32. Chijioke, O., & Münz, C. (2013, November 11). Dendritic cell derived cytokines in human natural killer cell differentiation and activation. Retrieved from https://www.ncbi.nlm.nih.gov/pmc/articles/PMC3822368/

33. Yang, Y.-ting T., Whiteman, M., & Gieseg, S. P. (2011, October 10). HOCl causes necrotic cell death in human monocyte derived macrophages through calcium dependent calpain activation. Retrieved from https://www.sciencedirect.com/science/article/pii/S0167488911002783

34. Baek S, Kim C S, Kim S B, Kim Y M, Kwon S W, Kim Y, Kim H, Lee H. Combination therapy of renal cell carcinoma or breast cancer patients with dendritic cell vaccine and IL-2: results from a phase I/II trial. Journal Of Translational Medicine [serial online]. January 2011;9(1):178-187.

35. Ying J, Yand X, Hao F, Xin X, Wu X, Pang Y. Dendritic cell vaccine treatment of advanced de novo colorectal cancer in renal transplant patients. Indian Journal Of Cancer [serial online]. July 2014;51(3):338-341.

36. Zhu H, Yang X, Pang Y, et al. Immune response, safety, and survival and quality of life outcomes for advanced colorectal cancer patients treated with dendritic cell vaccine and cytokine-induced killer cell therapy. Biomed Research International [serial online]. January 2014;:603871-603871 1p.

37. Shuo W, Yonghua W, Xinsheng W, et al. Silencing B7-H1 enhances the anti-tumor effect of bladder cancer antigen-loaded dendritic cell vaccine in vitro. Oncotargets & Therapy [serial online]. August 2014;7:1389-1395.

38. Katz T, Avivi I, Benyamini N, Rosenblatt J, Avigan D. Dendritic Cell Cancer Vaccines: From the Bench to the Bedside. Rambam Maimonides Medical Journal [serial online]. October 2014;5(4):1-11.

39. "Cancer Facts & Figures 2015." (2015): n. pag. American Cancer Society. Web.

40. Kobayashi M, Shimodaira S, Yonemitsu Y, et al. Prognostic factors related to add-on dendritic cell vaccines on patients with inoperable pancreatic cancer receiving chemotherapy: a multicenter analysis. Cancer Immunology, Immunotherapy [serial online]. August 2014;63(8):797-806.

41. Winter H, van den Engel N, Rüttinger D, et al. Active-specific immunotherapy for non-small cell lung cancer. Journal Of Thoracic Disease [serial online]. June 2011;3(2):105-114 10p.

42. Steele J, Rao A, Steven N, et al. Phase I/II trial of a dendritic cell vaccine transfected with DNA encoding melan A and gp100 for patients with metastatic melanoma. Gene Therapy [serial online]. June 2011;18(6):584-593.

43. Dobrovolskienė N, Strioga M, Gudlevičienė Ž, et al. Expression of tolerogenic potential-representing markers on clinical-grade therapeutic dendritic cell-based cancer vaccines. Acta Medica Lituanica [serial online]. October 2013;20(4):161-173.

44. Le, D. T., & Jaffee, E. M. (2012, July 15). Regulatory T-cell modulation using cyclophosphamide in vaccine approaches: a current perspective. Retrieved from https://www.ncbi.nlm.nih.gov/pmc/articles/PMC3399042/

45. Kalinski, P., Muthuswamy, R., & Urban, J. (2013, March). Dendritic cells in cancer immunotherapy: vaccines and combination immunotherapies. Retrieved from https://www.ncbi.nlm.nih.gov/pmc/articles/PMC6542562/

46. Saxena, M., & Bhardwaj, N. (2018, February). Re-Emergence of Dendritic Cell Vaccines for Cancer Treatment. Retrieved from https://www.ncbi.nlm.nih.gov/pmc/articles/PMC5823288/

47. Mastelic-Gavillet, B., Balint, K., Boudousquie, C., Gannon, P. O., & Kandalaft, L. E. (2019, April 11). Personalized Dendritic Cell Vaccines-Recent Breakthroughs and Encouraging Clinical Results. Retrieved from https://www.ncbi.nlm.nih.gov/pmc/articles/PMC6470191/

48. Lin T, Liang W, Yang N, et al. Rapamycin Promotes Mouse 4T1 Tumor Metastasis that Can Be Reversed by a Dendritic Cell-Based Vaccine. Plos ONE [serial online]. October 2015;10(10):1-21.

49. Gottschalk S, Yu F, Ji M, Kakarla S, Song X. A Vaccine That Co-Targets Tumor Cells and Cancer Associated Fibroblasts Results in Enhanced Antitumor Activity by Inducing Antigen Spreading. Plos ONE [serial online].

50. Wen C, Chen, H, Yang N, et al. Specific microtubule-depolymerizing agents augment efficacy of dendritic cell- based cancer vaccines. Journal Of Biomedical Science [serial online]. January 2011;18(1):44-58.

51. Chen H, Wang P, Yang N, et al. Shikonin induces immunogenic cell death in tumor cells and enhances dendritic cell-based cancer vaccine. Cancer Immunology, Immunotherapy: CII [serial online]. November 2012;61(11):1989-2002.

CHAPTER 12

1. Carter, I. (n.d.). The German 'Lightning War' Strategy Of The Second World War. Retrieved from https://www.iwm.org.uk/history/the-german-lightning-war-strategy-of-the-second-world-war

2. World War: After Dunkirk. (1940, June 17). Retrieved from http://content.time.com/time/subscriber/article/0,33009,789869,00.html

3. Rothman, L. (2017, May 25). World War II Dunkirk Evacuation: Read TIME's 1940 Report. Retrieved from https://time.com/4789230/dunkirk-france-world-war-ii-time-report/

4. Operation Dynamo at Dunkirk ends. (2010). Retrieved from https://www.history.com/this-day-in-history/dunkirk-evacuation-ends

5. Tzu, S. (2012). The Art of War. Chapter 11: The Nine Situations. Minneapolis, MN: Filiquarian Publishing.

6. Cannan, E. (1892). The Origin of the Law of Diminishing Returns, 1813-15. The Economic Journal. Volume 2 (5) pp. 53-69.

7. Mold, J. W., Hamm, R. M., & McCarthy, L. H. (2010). The law of diminishing returns in clinical medicine: how much risk reduction is enough? Retrieved from https://www.ncbi.nlm.nih.gov/pubmed/20453183

8. Berg JM, Tymoczko JL, Stryer L. (2002) Biochemistry. 5th edition. New York: W H Freeman.

9. Zheng, H.-C. (2017, July 6). The molecular mechanisms of chemoresistance in cancers. Retrieved from https://www.ncbi.nlm.nih.gov/pmc/articles/PMC5601792/

10. Yu, D. (1998, September). The role of oncogenes in drug resistance. Retrieved from https://www.ncbi.nlm.nih.gov/pmc/articles/PMC3449565/

11. Jasisinki-Bergner, S. Kielstein, H. (n.d.). Adipokines Regulate the Expression of Tumor-Relevant MicroRNAs. Retrieved from https://www.karger.com/Article/Fulltext/496625

12. Magee, P., Shi, L., & Garofalo, M. (2015, December). Role of microRNAs in chemoresistance. Retrieved from https://www.ncbi.nlm.nih.gov/pmc/articles/PMC4690999/

13. Chen, J., Zeng, F., Forrester, S. J., Eguchi, S., Zhang, M., Harris, R. C. (2016). Expression and Function of the Epidermal Growth Factor Receptor in Physiology and Disease. Physiological Reviews. 96:3, 1025-1069

14. Zandi, R., Larsen, A. B., Andersen, P., Stockhausen, M.-T., & Poulsen, H. S. (2007, October). Mechanisms for oncogenic activation of the epidermal growth factor receptor. Retrieved from https://www.ncbi.nlm.nih.gov/pubmed/17681753

15. Minder, P., Zajac, E., Quigley, J. P., & Deryugina, E. I. (2015, August). EGFR regulates the development and microarchitecture of intratumoral angiogenic vasculature capable of sustaining cancer cell intravasation. Retrieved from https://www.ncbi.nlm.nih.gov/pmc/articles/PMC4674488/

16. Mabe, N. W., Fox, D. B., Lupo, R., Decker, A. E., Phelps, S. N., Thompson, J. W., & Alvarez, J. V. (2018, October 1). Epigenetic silencing of tumor suppressor Par-4 promotes chemoresistance in recurrent breast cancer. Retrieved from https://www.jci.org/articles/view/99481

17. Rocha, C. R. R., Silva, M. M., Quinet, A., Cabral-Neto, J. B., & Menck, C. F. M. (2018, September 6). DNA repair pathways and cisplatin resistance: an intimate relationship. Retrieved from https://www.ncbi.nlm.nih.gov/pmc/articles/PMC6113849/

18. Li, X., Zhou, Y., Li, Y., Yang, L., Ma, Y., Peng, X., ... Li, H. (2019, September 9). Autophagy: A novel mechanism of chemoresistance in cancers. Retrieved from https://www.sciencedirect.com/science/article/pii/S075333221932373X

19. Moharil, R. B., Dive, A., Khandekar, S., & Bodhade, A. (2017). Cancer stem cells: An insight. Retrieved from https://www.ncbi.nlm.nih.gov/pmc/articles/PMC5763886/

20. Steinbichler, T. B., Dudás, J., Skvortsov, S., Ganswindt, U., Riechelmann, H., & Skvortsova, I.-I. (2019, March 30). Therapy resistance mediated by exosomes. Retrieved from https://www.ncbi.nlm.nih.gov/pmc/articles/PMC6441190/

21. Zhang, H.-G., & Grizzle, W. E. (2011, March 1). Exosomes and cancer: a newly described pathway of immune suppression. Retrieved from https://www.ncbi.nlm.nih.gov/pmc/articles/PMC3155407/

22. Kim, Ji, S., Kim, Soo, H., Seo, & Rok, Y. (2019, December 20). Understanding of ROS-Inducing Strategy in Anticancer Therapy. Retrieved from https://www.hindawi.com/journals/omcl/2019/5381692/

23. Kurutas, E.B. (2015). The importance of antioxidants which play the role in cellular response against oxidative/nitrosative stress: current state. Nutrition Journal.d 15 (71). https://doi.org/10.1186/s12937-016-0186-5

24. Saini, Nipun, Yang, & Xiaohe. (2017, October 7). Metformin as an anticancer agent: actions and mechanisms targeting cancer stem cells. Retrieved from https://academic.oup.com/abbs/article/50/2/133/4371596

25. West, J., & Newton, P. K. (2017, December 1). Chemotherapeutic Dose Scheduling Based on Tumor Growth Rates Provides a Case for Low-Dose Metronomic High-Entropy Therapies. Retrieved from https://www.ncbi.nlm.nih.gov/pmc/articles/PMC5712269/

26. Grosso, G. (2018, August 14). Effects of Polyphenol-Rich Foods on Human Health. Retrieved from https://www.ncbi.nlm.nih.gov/pmc/articles/PMC6115785/

27. Mileo, Maria, A., & Stefania. (2015, November 16). Polyphenols as Modulator of Oxidative Stress in Cancer Disease: New Therapeutic Strategies. Retrieved from https://www.hindawi.com/journals/omcl/2016/6475624/

28. Royston, K. J., & Tollefsbol, T. O. (2015, February 1). The Epigenetic Impact of Cruciferous Vegetables on Cancer Prevention. Retrieved from https://www.ncbi.nlm.nih.gov/pmc/articles/PMC4354933/

29. Snyder, V., Reed-Newman, T. C., Arnold, L., Thomas, S. M., & Anant, S. (2018, June 5). Cancer Stem Cell Metabolism and Potential Therapeutic Targets. Retrieved from https://www.ncbi.nlm.nih.gov/pmc/articles/PMC5996058/

30. Jampilek, J., Kos, J., & Kralova, K. (2019, February 19). Potential of Nanomaterial Applications in Dietary Supplements and Foods for Special Medical Purposes. Retrieved from https://www.ncbi.nlm.nih.gov/pmc/articles/PMC6409737/

31. Panda, A. K., Chakraborty, D., Sarkar, I., Khan, T., & Sa, G. (2017, March 31). New insights into therapeutic activity and anticancer properties of curcumin. Retrieved from https://www.ncbi.nlm.nih.gov/pmc/articles/PMC5386596/

32. Kaur, M., & Agarwal, R. (2007, November 1). Silymarin and epithelial cancer chemoprevention: how close we are to bedside? Retrieved from https://www.ncbi.nlm.nih.gov/pmc/articles/PMC2692696/

33. Singhal, K., Raj, N., Gupta, K., & Singh, S. (2017). Probable benefits of green tea with genetic implications. Retrieved from https://www.ncbi.nlm.nih.gov/pmc/articles/PMC5406788/

34. Katiyar, S. K., & Athar, M. (2013, July). Grape seeds: ripe for cancer chemoprevention. Retrieved from https://www.ncbi.nlm.nih.gov/pmc/articles/PMC3710656/

35. Weiskirchen, Sabine, Weiskirchen, & Ralf. (2016, July 11). Resveratrol: How Much Wine Do You Have to Drink to Stay Healthy? Retrieved from https://academic.oup.com/advances/article/7/4/706/4568690

36. Li, W., Liu, J., Fu, W. et al. (2018). 3-O-acetyl-11-keto-β-boswellic acid exerts anti-tumor effects in glioblastoma by arresting cell cycle at G2/M phase. Journal of Experimental Clinical Cancer Research. 37, 132. https://doi.org/10.1186/s13046-018-0805-4

37. Lü, J., Zhang, J., Jiang, C., Deng, Y., Özten, N., & Bosland, M. C. (2016). Cancer chemoprevention research with selenium in the post-SELECT era: Promises and challenges. Retrieved from https://www.ncbi.nlm.nih.gov/pmc/articles/PMC4822195/

38. Yildiz, A., Kaya, Y., & Tanriverdi, O. (2019, September). Effect of the Interaction Between Selenium and Zinc on DNA Repair in Association With Cancer Prevention. Retrieved from https://www.ncbi.nlm.nih.gov/pmc/articles/PMC6786808/

39. Dhawan, D. K., & Chadha, V. D. (2010, December). Zinc: a promising agent in dietary chemoprevention of cancer. Retrieved from https://www.ncbi.nlm.nih.gov/pmc/articles/PMC3102454/

40. Vučetić, M., Cormerais, Y., Parks, S. K., & Pouysségur, J. (2017, December 21). The Central Role of Amino Acids in Cancer Redox Homeostasis: Vulnerability Points of the Cancer Redox Code. Retrieved from https://www.ncbi.nlm.nih.gov/pmc/articles/PMC5742588/

41. Lee, J. Y., Sim, T.-B., Lee, J.-E., & Na, H.-K. (2017, July). Chemopreventive and Chemotherapeutic Effects of Fish Oil derived Omega-3 Polyunsaturated Fatty Acids on Colon Carcinogenesis. Retrieved from https://www.ncbi.nlm.nih.gov/pmc/articles/PMC5539209/

42. Shimizu, Y. et al. (2019). Amelioration of Radiation Enteropathy by Dietary Supplementation With Reduced Coenzyme Q10. Advances in Radiation Oncology, Volume 4 (2) pp. 237 – 245.

43. Giammanco, M. (n.d.). Vitamin D in cancer chemoprevention. Retrieved from https://www.tandfonline.com/doi/full/10.3109/13880209.2014.988274

44. The Role of Cyclooxgenase-2 (COX-2) in Breast Cancer, and Implications of COX-2 Inhibition. (2002). European Journal of Surgical Oncology (EJSO), 28(1), 96. doi: 10.1053/ejso.2001.1227

45. Cechin, S. R., & Buchwald, P. (2014, July). Effects of representative glucocorticoids on TNFα- and CD40L-induced NF-κB activation in sensor cells. Retrieved from https://www.ncbi.nlm.nih.gov/pmc/articles/PMC4049353/

46. McCarty, M. F., & Block, K. I. (2006, September). Preadministration of high-dose salicylates, suppressors of NF-kappaB activation, may increase the chemosensitivity of many cancers: an example of proapoptotic signal modulation therapy. Retrieved from https://www.ncbi.nlm.nih.gov/pubmed/16880431

47. McCarty, M. F., Barroso-Aranda, J., & Contreras, F. (2010, May). Practical strategies for suppressing hypoxia-inducible factor activity in cancer therapy. Retrieved from https://www.ncbi.nlm.nih.gov/pubmed/20089365

48. Raina, K., Agarwal, C., & Agarwal, R. (2013, March). Effect of silibinin in human colorectal cancer cells: targeting the activation of NF-κB signaling. Retrieved from https://www.ncbi.nlm.nih.gov/pmc/articles/PMC3563833/

CHAPTER 13

1. Lohnes, K., & Sommerville, D. (2019, July 5). Battle of Thermopylae. Retrieved from https://www.britannica.com/event/Battle-of-Thermopylae-Greek-history-480-BC.

2. Nunnari, G., (Producer), Canton, M. (Producer) & Snyder, Z. (Director). (2007). 300 [Motion Picture]. USA: Legendary Pictures.

3. Tzu, S. (2012). The Art of War. Minneapolis, MN: Filiquarian Publishing.

4. Jemal, A., Ward, E. M., Johnson, C. J., Cronin, K. A., Ma, J., Ryerson, B., & Weir, H. K. (2017). Annual Report to the Nation on the Status of Cancer, 1975-2014, Featuring Survival. Retrieved from https://www.ncbi.nlm.nih.gov/pmc/articles/PMC5409140/.

5. Hiom, S. C. (2015). Diagnosing cancer earlier: reviewing the evidence for improving cancer survival. Retrieved from https://www.ncbi.nlm.nih.gov/pmc/articles/PMC4385969/.

6. Miglioretti, D. L., Lange, J., van den Broek, J. J., Lee, C. I., van Ravesteyn, N. T., Ritley, D., & Hubbard, R. A. (2016). Radiation-Induced Breast Cancer Incidence and Mortality From Digital Mammography Screening: A Modeling Study. Retrieved from https://www.ncbi.nlm.nih.gov/pmc/articles/PMC4878445/.

7. Pilevarzadeh, M. (2016, September). Women's Perspective of Breast Self-examination. Retrieved from https://www.ncbi.nlm.nih.gov/pmc/articles/PMC5080410/.

8. Hackshaw, A. K., & Paul, E. A. (2003, April 1). Breast self-examination and death from breast cancer: a meta-analysis. Retrieved from https://www.nature.com/articles/6600847.

9. Sood, R., Rositch, A. F., Shakoor, D., Ambinder, E., Pool, K. L., & Pollack, E. (2019, August 27). Ultrasound for Breast Cancer Detection Globally: A Systematic Review and Meta-Analysis. Retrieved from https://ascopubs.org/doi/full/10.1200/JGO.19.00127.

10. Rebolj, M., Assi, V., Brentnall, A., Parmar, D., & Duffy, S. W. (2018, May 8). Addition of ultrasound to mammography in the case of dense breast tissue: systematic review and meta-analysis. Retrieved from https://www.nature.com/articles/s41416-018-0080-3.

11. Lee, S. Y., Park, H. J., Kim, M. S., Rho, M. H., & Han, C. H. (2018, November 21). An initial experience with the use of whole body MRI for cancer screening and regular health checks. Retrieved from https://www.ncbi.nlm.nih.gov/pmc/articles/PMC6248944/.

12. Jones, D., Friend, C., Dreher, A., Allgar, V., & Macleod, U. (2018, June 2). The diagnostic test accuracy of rectal examination for prostate cancer diagnosis in symptomatic patients: a systematic review. Retrieved from https://www.ncbi.nlm.nih.gov/pmc/articles/PMC5985061/.

13. Li, D. (2018). Recent advances in colorectal cancer screening. Retrieved from https://www.ncbi.nlm.nih.gov/pmc/articles/PMC6160607/.

14. Bénard, F., Barkun, A. N., Martel, M., & von Renteln, D. (2018). Systematic review of colorectal cancer screening guidelines for average-risk adults: Summarizing the current global recommendations. Retrieved from https://www.ncbi.nlm.nih.gov/pmc/articles/PMC5757117/.

15. Kim, S. Y., Kim, H.-S., & Park, H. J. (2019, January 14). Adverse events related to colonoscopy: Global trends and future challenges. Retrieved from https://www.ncbi.nlm.nih.gov/pmc/articles/PMC6337013/.

16. Neal, R. D., Barham, A., Bongard, E., Edwards, R. T., Fitzgibbon, J., Griffiths, G., ... Hurt, C. N. (2017, January). Immediate chest X-ray for patients at risk of lung cancer presenting in primary care: randomised controlled feasibility trial. Retrieved from https://www.ncbi.nlm.nih.gov/pmc/articles/PMC5294478/.

17. Powell, A. C., Mirhadi, A. J., Loy, B. A., Happe, L. E., Long, J. W., Kren, E. M., & Gupta, A. K. (n.d.). Presentation at computed tomography (CT) scan of the thorax and first year diagnostic and treatment utilization among patients diagnosed with lung cancer. Retrieved from https://journals.plos.org/plosone/article?id=10.1371/journal.pone.0181319.

18. Pauwels, E. K. J., Coumou, A. W., Kostkiewicz, M., & Kairemo, K. (2013). [^{18}F]fluoro-2-deoxy-d-glucose positron emission tomography/computed tomography imaging in oncology: initial staging and evaluation of cancer therapy. Retrieved from https://www.ncbi.nlm.nih.gov/pmc/articles/PMC5586772/.

19. Griffeth, L. K. (2005, October). Use of PET/CT scanning in cancer patients: technical and practical considerations. Retrieved from https://www.ncbi.nlm.nih.gov/pmc/articles/PMC1255942/.

20. Hu, C., Liu, C.-P., Cheng, J.-S., Chiu, Y.-L., Chan, H.-P., & Peng, N.-J. (2016, November). Application of whole-body FDG-PET for cancer screening in a cohort of hospital employees. Retrieved from https://www.ncbi.nlm.nih.gov/pmc/articles/PMC5591093/.

21. Chien, J., & Poole, E. M. (2017). Ovarian Cancer Prevention, Screening, and Early Detection: Report From the 11th Biennial Ovarian Cancer Research Symposium. Retrieved from https://www.ncbi.nlm.nih.gov/pmc/articles/PMC6154781/.

22. Nagpal, M., Singh, S., Singh, P., Chauhan, P., & Zaidi, M. A. (2016). Tumor markers: A diagnostic tool. Retrieved from https://www.ncbi.nlm.nih.gov/pmc/articles/PMC5242068/.

23. Etzioni, Ruth, Penson, F., D., Legler, M., J., ... J., E. (2002, July 3). Overdiagnosis Due to Prostate-Specific Antigen Screening: Lessons From U.S. Prostate Cancer Incidence Trends. Retrieved from https://academic.oup.com/jnci/article/94/13/981/2519795.

24. Shyamala, K., Girish, H. C., & Murgod, S. (2014, January). Risk of tumor cell seeding through biopsy and aspiration cytology. Retrieved from https://www.ncbi.nlm.nih.gov/pmc/articles/PMC4015162/.

25. How Cancer Is Diagnosed. (n.d.). Retrieved from https://www.cancer.gov/about-cancer/diagnosis-staging/diagnosis.

26. Gaya, A., Giakoustidis, A., Winslet, M., & Mudan, S. (2015, December 21). Tumor Biology: Is It Time to Redefine Unresectability? An Extraordinary Case of Gastroesophageal Junctional Adenocarcinoma. Retrieved from https://www.ncbi.nlm.nih.gov/pmc/articles/PMC4725854/.

27. Survival Rates for Kidney Cancer. (n.d.). Retrieved from https://www.cancer.org/cancer/kidney-cancer/detection-diagnosis-staging/survival-rates.html.

28. Reyes-Botero, G., Mokhtari, K., Martin-Duverneuil, N., Delattre, J.-Y., & Laigle-Donadey, F. (2012). Adult brainstem gliomas. Retrieved from https://www.ncbi.nlm.nih.gov/pmc/articles/PMC3316925/.

29. Curigliano, G., Criscitiello, C., Esposito, A., Fumagalli, L., Gelao, L., Locatelli, M., ... Goldhirsch, A. (2013, September). Best management of locally advanced inoperable breast cancer. Retrieved from https://www.ncbi.nlm.nih.gov/pmc/articles/PMC4041552/.

30. Catena, F., De Simone, B., Coccolini, F. et al. (2019). Bowel obstruction: a narrative review for all physicians. World J Emerg Surg 14, 20. doi:10.1186/s13017-019-0240-7

31. Schorge, J. O., McCann, C., & Del Carmen, M. G. (2010). Surgical debulking of ovarian cancer: what difference does it make? Retrieved from https://www.ncbi.nlm.nih.gov/pmc/articles/PMC3046749/.

32. Reyal, F., Hamy, A. S., & Piccart, M. J. (2018, May 17). Neoadjuvant treatment: the future of patients with breast cancer. Retrieved from https://www.ncbi.nlm.nih.gov/pmc/articles/PMC5976132/.

33. Lee, Y. S., Lee, J.-C., Yang, S. Y., Kim, J., & Hwang, J.-H. (2019, October 30). Neoadjuvant therapy versus upfront surgery in resectable pancreatic cancer according to intention-to-treat and per-protocol analysis: A systematic review and meta-analysis. Retrieved from https://www.nature.com/articles/s41598-019-52167-9.

34. National Cancer Institute. (Ed.). (n.d.). Cancer Staging. Retrieved from https://www.cancer.gov/about-cancer/diagnosis-staging/staging

35. Saraee, A., Vahedian-Ardakani, J., Saraee, E. et al. (2015). Whipple procedure: a review of a 7-year clinical experience in a referral center for hepatobiliary and pancreas diseases. World Journal of Surgical Oncology. 13 (98). https://doi.org/10.1186/s12957-015-0523-8

36. Brouwer, N. P. M., Bos, A. C. R. K., Lemmens, V. E. P. P., Tanis, P. J., Hugen, N., Nagtegaal, I. D., ... Verhoeven, R. H. A. (2018). An overview of 25 years of incidence, treatment and outcome of colorectal cancer patients. Retrieved from https://www.ncbi.nlm.nih.gov/pmc/articles/PMC6282554/

37. NCI Dictionary of Cancer Terms. (n.d.). Retrieved from https://www.cancer.gov/publications/dictionaries/cancer-terms/search?contains=false&q=advance+staged+cancer

38. NCI Dictionary of Cancer Terms. (n.d.). Retrieved from https://www.cancer.gov/publications/dictionaries/cancer-terms/def/advanced-cancer

39. Cho, H., Mariotto, A. B., Schwartz, L. M., Luo, J., & Woloshin, S. (2014, November). When do changes in cancer survival mean progress? The insight from population incidence and mortality. Retrieved from https://www.ncbi.nlm.nih.gov/pmc/articles/PMC4841163/

40. Browse the SEER Cancer Statistics Review 1975-2016. (n.d.). Retrieved from https://seer.cancer.gov/csr/1975_2016/browse_csr.php

41. Contreras, F., McCarty, M. (n.d.). Patients with Metastatic Cancer Treated with Integrative Regulatory Therapies . Retrieved February 17, 2020, from https://www.townsendletter.com/AugSept2012/metastatic0812.html

CHAPTER 14

1. Four Humors - And there's the humor of it: Shakespeare and the four humors. (2013). Retrieved from https://www.nlm.nih.gov/exhibition/shakespeare/fourhumors.html.
2. Lagay, F. (2002, July 1). The Legacy of Humoral Medicine. Retrieved from https://journalofethics.ama-assn.org/article/legacy-humoral-medicine/2002-07.
3. Howart, E. (2002, June 4). Mood differences between the four Galen personality types: choleric, sanguine, phlegmatic, melancholic. Retrieved from https://www.sciencedirect.com/science/article/abs/pii/019188698890044X.
4. Klein, D. N., Kotov, R., & Bufferd, S. J. (2011). Personality and depression: explanatory models and review of the evidence. Retrieved from https://www.ncbi.nlm.nih.gov/pmc/articles/PMC3518491/.
5. Kennedy, Daniel. (Producer & Director). (2020). Healthy Long Life [Documentary Series]. United States: Eagle's Flight Studio.
6. Höckel M, Vaupel P.(2001). Tumor hypoxia: definitions and current clinical, biologic, and molecular aspects. J Natl Cancer Inst. 93(4):266-76.
7. Buffa FM, Harris AL, West CM, Miller CJ. Large meta-analysis of multiple cancers reveals a common, compact and highly prognostic hypoxia metagene. Br J Cancer. 2010 Jan 19;102(2):428-35. Erratum in: Br J Cancer. 2010 Sep 7;103(6):929.
8. Parks S, Mazure N, Counillon L, Pouysségur J. Hypoxia promotes tumor cell survival in acidic conditions by preserving ATP levels. Journal of Cellular Physiology [serial online]. September 2013;228(9):1854-1862.
9. Elvis AM. Ekta JS. (2011) Ozone therapy: A clinical review. Journal of Natural Science Biology & Medicine. 2(1):66-70.
10. Cassileth B. (2009) Oxygen therapies. Oncology (Williston Park). 23(13):1182.
11. Guanche D, Zamora Z, Gonzales R, et al. Effect of Ozone/oxygen mixture on systemic oxidative stress and organic damage. Toxicology Mechanisms and Methods [serial online]. January 2010;20(1):25-30.

12. Clavo, Bernardino, Juan L. Pérez, Laura López, Gerardo Suárez, Marta Lloret, Victor Rodríguez, David Macías, Maite Santana, María A. Hernández, Roberto Martín-Oliva, and Francisco Robaina. "Ozone Therapy for Tumor Oxygenation: A Pilot Study." Evidence-based Complementary and Alternative Medicine. Oxford University Press, n.d. Web. 12 Oct. 2015.Bocci V., Larini A., Micheli V. (2005). Restoration of normoxia by Ozone therapy may control neoplastic growth: A review and a working hypothesis. Journal of Alternative and Complementary Medicine. 11 (2): pp 257-265.

13. Burke FJ.(2012). Ozone and caries: a review of the literature. Dent Update. 39(4):271-2, 275-8. European Cooperation of Medical Ozone Societies EUROCOOP (Ärztliche Gesellschaft für Ozon-Anwendung in Prävention und Therapie). Information for patients.

14. Sagai M., Bocci V. (2011). Med Gas Res. 2011 Dec 20;1:29. Mechanisms of action involved in Ozone therapy: Is healing induced via a mild oxidative stress? Medical Gas Research. 1 (1). Article Number: 29.

15. Bocci V.A.(2006). Scientific and medical aspects of Ozone therapy. State of the Art. Archives of Medical Research. 37 (4) (pp 425-435).

16. FalK SJ, War R, Bleehen NM. The influence of carbogen breathing on tumor tissue oxygenation in man evaluated by computerized pO2 histography. British Journal of Cancer. 1992;66:919-24.

17. Bucci B., Cannizzaro A., Brunetti E., Martinelli M. Ozone treatment inhibits proliferation in human neuroblastoma SK-N-SH cells. Rivista Italiana di Ossigeno-Ozonoterapia. 5 (2) (pp 85-92), 2006.

18. Sweet F., Kao M., Lee S., Hagar W., Sweet W. Ozone selectively inhibits growth of human cancer cells. Science. 209 (4459) (pp931-993), 1980.

19. Schulz S, Haussler U, Mandic R, Heverhagen JT, Neubauer A, Dunne AA et al. Treatment with Ozone/oxygen-pneumoperitoneum results in complete remission of rabbit squamous cell carcinomas. Int J Cancer 2008; 122(10):2360-2367.

20. Cannizzaro A, Verga Falzacappa C, Martinelli M, Misiti S, Brunetti E, Bucci B. O(2/3) exposure inhibits cell progression affecting cyclin B1/cdk1 activity in SK-N-SH while induces apoptosis in SK-N-DZ neuroblastoma cells. Journal of Cellular Physiology [serial online]. October 2007;213(1):115-125.

21. Menéndez S, Cepero J, Borrego L. Ozone therapy in cancer treatment: state of the art. Ozone: Science & Engineering [serial online]. November 2008;30(6):398-404.

22. Clavo B, Ruiz A, Lloret M, López L, Suárez G, Macías D, Rodríguez V, Hernández MA, Martín-Oliva R, Quintero S, Cuyás JM, Robaina F. Adjuvant Ozone therapy in advanced head and neck tumors: a comparative study. Evid Based Complement Alternat Med. 2004 Dec;1(3):321-325. Epub 2004 Oct 16.

23. Zanker KS, Kroczek R. In vitro synergistic activity of 5-fluorouracil with low-dose Ozone against a chemoresistant tumor cell line and fresh human tumor cells. Chemotherapy 1990; 36(2):147-154.

24. Liu Q, He X. Clinical evaluation of sequential medical Ozone therapy for the primary liver cancer patients after trans-arterial chemoembolization. International Journal of Ozone Therapy [serial online]. April 2012;11(1):53-55.

25. Parkhisenko I, Bil'chenko SV.(2003). [The Ozone therapy in patients with mechanical jaundice of tumorous genesis]. Vestn Khir Im I I Grek 162(5):85-87.

26. Clavo B., Santana-Rodriguez N., Llontop P., et al. "Ozone Therapy in the Management of Persistent Radiation-Induced Rectal Bleeding in Prostate Cancer Patients," Evidence-Based Complementary and Alternative Medicine, vol. 2015, Article ID 480369, 7 pages, 2015.

27. Sonkin, P. L., Chen, L. E., Seaber, A. V., & Hatchell, D. L. (1992, June). Vasodilator action of Pentoxifylline on microcirculation of rat cremaster muscle. Retrieved from https://www.ncbi.nlm.nih.gov/pubmed/1595940.s

28. Hood SC, Moher D, Barber GG. Management of intermittent claudication with Pentoxifylline: meta-analysis of randomized controlled trials. CMAJ 1996 October 15;155(8):1053-9.

29. Salhiyyah K, Senanayake E, Abdel-Hadi M, Booth A, Michaels JA. Pentoxifylline for intermittent claudication. Cochrane Database Syst Rev 2012;1:CD005262.

30. Curjuric I, Imboden M, Adam M et al. Serum bilirubin is associated with lung function in a Swiss general population sample. Eur Respir J 2014 May;43(5):1278-88.

31. Ott E, Lechner H, Fazekas F. Hemorheological effects of Pentoxifylline on disturbed flow behavior of blood in patients with cerebrovascular insufficiency. Eur Neurol 1983;22 Suppl 1:105-7.

32. Strano A, Davi G, Avellone G, Novo S, Pinto A. Double-blind, crossover study of the clinical efficacy and the hemorheological effects of Pentoxifylline in patients with occlusive arterial disease of the lower limbs. Angiology 1984 July;35(7):459-66.

33. Perego MA, Sergio G, Artale F, Giunti P, Danese C. Haemorrheological improvement by Pentoxifylline in patients with peripheral arterial occlusive disease. Curr Med Res Opin 1986;10(2):135-8.

34. Soria J, Giovannangeli ML, Jolchine IE, Chassoux G. Pentoxifylline, fibrinogen and leukocytes. Blood Coagul Fibrinolysis 1990 October;1(4-5):485-7.

35. Fossat C, Fabre D, Alimi Y et al. Leukocyte activation study during occlusive arterial disease of the lower limb: effect of Pentoxifylline infusion. J Cardiovasc Pharmacol 1995;25 Suppl 2:S96-100.

36. Armstrong M, Jr., Needham D, Hatchell DL, Nunn RS. Effect of Pentoxifylline on the flow of polymorphonuclear leukocytes through a model capillary. Angiology 1990 April;41(4):253-62.

37. Munn LL. Aberrant vascular architecture in tumors and its importance in drug-based therapies. Drug Discov Today 2003 May 1;8(9):396-403.

38. Song CW, Hasegawa T, Kwon HC, Lyons JC, Levitt SH. Increase in tumor oxygenation and radiosensitivity caused by Pentoxifylline. Radiat Res 1992 May;130(2):205-10.

39. Lee I, Boucher Y, Demhartner TJ, Jain RK. Changes in tumour blood flow, oxygenation and interstitial fluid pressure induced by Pentoxifylline. Br J Cancer 1994 March;69(3):492-6.

40. Song CW, Makepeace CM, Griffin RJ et al. Increase in tumor blood flow by Pentoxifylline. Int J Radiat Oncol Biol Phys 1994 June 15;29(3):433-7.

41. Honess DJ, Andrews MS, Ward R, Bleehen NM. Pentoxifylline increases RIF-1 tumour pO2 in a manner compatible with its ability to increase relative tumour perfusion. Acta Oncol 1995;34(3):385-9.

42. Kelleher DK, Thews O, Vaupel P. Regional perfusion and oxygenation of tumors upon methylxanthine derivative administration. Int J Radiat Oncol Biol Phys 1998 November 1;42(4):861-4.

43. Collingridge DR, Rockwell S. Pentoxifylline improves the oxygenation and radiation response of BA1112 rat rhabdomyosarcomas and EMT6 mouse mammary carcinomas. Int J Cancer 2000 October 20;90(5):256-64.

44. Lee I, Biaglow JE, Lee J, Cho MJ. Physiological mechanisms of radiation sensitization by Pentoxifylline. Anticancer Res 2000 November;20(6B):4605-9.

45. Bennewith KL, Durand RE. Drug-induced alterations in tumour perfusion yield increases in tumour cell radiosensitivity. Br J Cancer 2001 November 16;85(10):1577-84.

46. Sibtain A, Hill S, Goodchild K, Shah N, Saunders M, Hoskin PJ. The modification of human tumour blood flow using Pentoxifylline, nicotinamide and carbogen. Radiother Oncol 2002 January;62(1):69-76.

47. Zywietz F, Bohm L, Sagowski C, Kehrl W. Pentoxifylline enhances tumor oxygenation and radiosensitivity in rat rhabdomyosarcomas during continuous hyperfractionated irradiation. Strahlenther Onkol 2004 May;180(5):306-14.

48. Tanaka, Y., Saihara, Y., Izumotani, K., & Nakamura, H. (2019, January 9). Daily ingestion of alkaline electrolyzed water containing hydrogen influences human health, including gastrointestinal symptoms. Retrieved from https://www.ncbi.nlm.nih.gov/pmc/articles/PMC6352572/.

49. Zhang, H. (2017, March). Will cancer cells be defeated by sodium bicarbonate? Retrieved from https://www.ncbi.nlm.nih.gov/pmc/articles/PMC5954837/.

50. Robey, I. F., & Nesbit, L. A. (2013). Investigating mechanisms of alkalinization for reducing primary breast tumor invasion. Retrieved from https://www.ncbi.nlm.nih.gov/pmc/articles/PMC3722989/.

51. Griffiths, J. R. (1991, September). Are cancer cells acidic? Retrieved from https://www.ncbi.nlm.nih.gov/pmc/articles/PMC1977628/?page=2.

52. Yan, D., Cui, H., Zhu, W., Talbot, A., Zhang, L. G., Sherman, J. H., & Keidar, M. (2017, September 7). The Strong Cell-based Hydrogen Peroxide Generation Triggered by Cold Atmospheric Plasma. Retrieved from https://www.nature.com/articles/s41598-017-11480-x

53. Aykin-Burns, N., Ahmad, I. M., Zhu, Y., Oberley, L. W., & Spitz, D. R. (2009, February 15). Increased levels of superoxide and H2O2 mediate the differential susceptibility of cancer cells versus normal cells to glucose deprivation. Retrieved from https://www.ncbi.nlm.nih.gov/pmc/articles/PMC2678564/

54. Ríos-Arrabal, S., Artacho-Cordón, F., León, J., Román-Marinetto, E., Del Mar Salinas-Asensio, M., Calvente, I., & Núñez, M. I. (2013, August 27). Involvement of free radicals in breast cancer. Retrieved from https://www.ncbi.nlm.nih.gov/pmc/articles/PMC3765596/

55. Puppo, A., & Halliwell, B. (1988, January 1). Formation of hydroxyl radicals from hydrogen peroxide in the presence of iron. Is haemoglobin a biological Fenton reagent? Retrieved from https://www.ncbi.nlm.nih.gov/pmc/articles/PMC1148683/

56. Ahmed K, Zaidi S. Treating cancer with heat: hyperthermia as promising strategy to enhance apoptosis. JPMA. The Journal Of The Pakistan Medical Association [serial online]. April 2013;63(4):504-508.

57. Qin S, Xu C, Ren H, et al. Hyperthermia induces apoptosis by targeting Survivin in esophageal cancer. Oncology Reports [serial online]. November 2015;34(5):2656-2664.

58. Mantso, T., Vasileiadis, S., Anestopoulos, I., Voulgaridou, G. P., Lampri, E., Botaitis, S., ... Panayiotidis, M. I. (2018, July 16). Hyperthermia induces therapeutic effectiveness and potentiates adjuvant therapy with non-targeted and targeted drugs in an in vitro model of human malignant melanoma. Retrieved from https://www.ncbi.nlm.nih.gov/pmc/articles/PMC6048057/

59. McCarty, M. F., & Contreras, F. (2014, September 16). Increasing Superoxide Production and the Labile Iron Pool in Tumor Cells may Sensitize Them to Extracellular Ascorbate. Retrieved from https://www.ncbi.nlm.nih.gov/pmc/articles/PMC4165285/

CHAPTER 15

1. Dylan, B. (1967). All Along The Watchtower. John Wesley Harding. Columbia Studio A. Nashville, TN.
2. Hendrix, J. (1968). All Along The Watchtower. Electric Ladyland. Olympic Stadium, London, UK. Record Plant & Mayfair, New York, NY. Rolling Stone. (2019, July 29).
3. Rolling Stone. (2019, July 29). 500 Greatest Songs of All Time. Retrieved from https://www.rollingstone.com/music/music-lists/500-greatest-songs-of-all-time-151127/.
4. Holy Bible Modern English Version. (2014). Isaiah 21:5-9. Lake Mary, FL: Charisma House.
5. Understanding Laboratory Tests Fact Sheet. (n.d.). Retrieved from https://www.cancer.gov/about-cancer/diagnosis-staging/understanding-lab-tests-fact-sheet.
6. Brady, A. P. (2017, February). Error and discrepancy in radiology: inevitable or avoidable? Retrieved from https://www.ncbi.nlm.nih.gov/pmc/articles/PMC5265198/.
7. Reiner, R. (Producer & Director). (2007). The Bucket List [Motion Picture]. USA: Castle Rock Entertainment.
8. Kessler, D., & Kübler-Ross, E. (n.d.). Retrieved from https://grief.com/the-five-stages-of-grief/.
9. Frankl, V. E., & Lasch, H. (1962). Mans search for meaning: an introduction to logotheraphy. London: Hodder and Stoughton.
10. Ross, M., Stoll, S. (2016). Change: Transforming Yourself and Your Body into the Person You Want to Be. Square One Publishers.
11. Contreras, F., Kennedy, D. (2013). 50 Critical Cancer Answers. Sydney:Authentic Media.
12. Sherpa. (n.d.). Retrieved from https://www.merriam-webster.com/dictionary/Sherpa.
13. Shanmugam, M. K., Kannaiyan, R., Sethi, G. Targeting Cell Signaling and Apoptotic Pathways by Dietary Agents: Role in the Prevention and Treatment of Cancer. Nutrition & Cancer, S1(63.2):1616-173.

14. Malaguti-Boyle, M. (2014). Can Spices Modify the Cancer Cell Signaling Pathway? Journal of the Australian Traditional-Medicine Society, 20(1), 32–37.

15. Meyts, P. D. (2016, April 27). The Insulin Receptor and Its Signal Transduction Network. Retrieved from https://www.ncbi.nlm.nih.gov/books/NBK378978/.

16. Fürstenberger, G., & Senn, H.-J. (2002, May). Insulin-like growth factors and cancer. Retrieved from https://www.ncbi.nlm.nih.gov/pubmed/12067807.

17. Allen, N. E., Appleby, P. N., Davey, G. K., Kaaks, R., Rinaldi, S., & Key, T. J. (2002, November). The associations of diet with serum insulin-like growth factor I and its main binding proteins in 292 women meat-eaters, vegetarians, and vegans. Retrieved from https://www.ncbi.nlm.nih.gov/pubmed/12433724.

18. McCarty MF, Barroso-Aranda J, Contreras F. (2009, Febraury). The low-methionine content of vegan diets may make methionine restriction feasible as a life extension strategy. Med Hypotheses. 72(2):125-8.

19. Richardson, J. L., Shelton, D. R., Krailo, M., Levine, A. M. (1990, February). The effect of compliance with treatment on survival among patients with hematologic malignancies. Journal of Clinical Oncology. 8, (2) pp. 356-364.

20. Hebert-Croteau, N., Brisson J., Latreille, J., Rivard, M., Abdelaziz, N., Martin, G. (2004, September). Compliance With Consensus Recommendations for Systemic Therapy Is Associated With Improved Survival of Women With Node-Negative Breast Cancer. Journal of Clinical Oncology. 22(18) pp. 3685-3693.

21. Moharil, R. B., Dive, A., Khandekar, S., & Bodhade, A. (2017). Cancer stem cells: An insight. Retrieved from https://www.ncbi.nlm.nih.gov/pmc/articles/PMC5763886/.

22. Zhou G, Myers R, Li Y et al. Role of AMP-activated protein kinase in mechanism of Metformin action. J Clin Invest 2001 October;108(8):1167-74.

23. Musi N, Hirshman MF, Nygren J et al. Metformin increases AMP-activated protein kinase activity in skeletal muscle of subjects with type 2 diabetes. Diabetes 2002 July;51(7):2074-81.

24. An H, He L. Current understanding of Metformin effect on the control of hyperglycemia in diabetes. J Endocrinol 2016 March;228(3):R97-R106.

25. Decensi A, Puntoni M, Goodwin P et al. Metformin and cancer risk in diabetic patients: a systematic review and meta-analysis. Cancer Prev Res (Phila) 2010 November;3(11):1451-61.

26. Zhang ZJ, Zheng ZJ, Kan H et al. Reduced risk of colorectal cancer with Metformin therapy in patients with type 2 diabetes: a meta-analysis. Diabetes Care 2011 October;34(10):2323-8.

27. Noto H, Goto A, Tsujimoto T, Noda M. Cancer risk in diabetic patients treated with Metformin: a systematic review and meta-analysis. PLoS ONE 2012;7(3):e33411.

28. Soranna D, Scotti L, Zambon A et al. Cancer risk associated with use of Metformin and sulfonylurea in type 2 diabetes: a meta-analysis. Oncologist 2012;17(6):813-22.

29. Singh S, Singh PP, Singh AG, Murad MH, Sanchez W. Anti-diabetic medications and the risk of hepatocellular cancer: a systematic review and meta-analysis. Am J Gastroenterol 2013 June;108(6):881-91.

30. Franciosi M, Lucisano G, Lapice E, Strippoli GF, Pellegrini F, Nicolucci A. Metformin therapy and risk of cancer in patients with type 2 diabetes: systematic review. PLoS ONE 2013;8(8):e71583.

31. Singh S, Singh H, Singh PP, Murad MH, Limburg PJ. Antidiabetic medications and the risk of colorectal cancer in patients with diabetes mellitus: a systematic review and meta-analysis. Cancer Epidemiol Biomarkers Prev 2013 December;22(12):2258-68.

32. Wang Z, Lai ST, Xie L et al. Metformin is associated with reduced risk of pancreatic cancer in patients with type 2 diabetes mellitus: a systematic review and meta-analysis. Diabetes Res Clin Pract 2014 October;106(1):19-26.

33. Zhang ZJ, Bi Y, Li S et al. Reduced risk of lung cancer with Metformin therapy in diabetic patients: a systematic review and meta-analysis. Am J Epidemiol 2014 July 1;180(1):11-4.

34. Yu H, Yin L, Jiang X et al. Effect of Metformin on cancer risk and treatment outcome of prostate cancer: a meta-analysis of epidemiological observational studies. PLoS ONE 2014;9(12):e116327.

35. Zhu N, Zhang Y, Gong YI, He J, Chen X. Metformin and lung cancer risk of patients with type 2 diabetes mellitus: A meta-analysis. Biomed Rep 2015 March;3(2):235-41.

36. Wu L, Zhu J, Prokop LJ, Murad MH. Pharmacologic Therapy of Diabetes and Overall Cancer Risk and Mortality: A Meta-Analysis of 265 Studies. Sci Rep 2015;5:10147.

37. Yang T, Yang Y, Liu S. Association between Metformin Therapy and Breast Cancer Incidence and Mortality: Evidence from a Meta-Analysis. J Breast Cancer 2015 September;18(3):264-70.

38. Zhang ZJ, Li S. The prognostic value of Metformin for cancer patients with concurrent diabetes: a systematic review and meta-analysis. Diabetes Obes Metab 2014 August;16(8):707-10.

39. Yin M, Zhou J, Gorak EJ, Quddus F. Metformin is associated with survival benefit in cancer patients with concurrent type 2 diabetes: a systematic review and meta-analysis. Oncologist 2013;18(12):1248-55.

40. Mei ZB, Zhang ZJ, Liu CY et al. Survival benefits of Metformin for colorectal cancer patients with diabetes: a systematic review and meta-analysis. PLoS ONE 2014;9(3):e91818.

41. Raval AD, Thakker D, Vyas A, Salkini M, Madhavan S, Sambamoorthi U. Impact of Metformin on clinical outcomes among men with prostate cancer: a systematic review and meta-analysis. Prostate Cancer Prostatic Dis 2015 June;18(2):110-21.

42. Hwang IC, Park SM, Shin D, Ahn HY, Rieken M, Shariat SF. Metformin association with lower prostate cancer recurrence in type 2 diabetes: a systematic review and meta-analysis. Asian Pac J Cancer Prev 2015;16(2):595-600.

43. Zhang JW, Sun Q. Metformin may improve the prognosis of patients with pancreatic cancer. Asian Pac J Cancer Prev 2015;16(9):3937-40.

44. Stopsack KH, Ziehr DR, Rider JR, Giovannucci EL. Metformin and prostate cancer mortality: a meta-analysis. Cancer Causes Control 2016 January;27(1):105-13.

45. McCarty MF. mTORC1 activity as a determinant of cancer risk--rationalizing the cancer-preventive effects of adiponectin, Metformin, rapamycin, and low-protein vegan diets. Med Hypotheses 2011 October;77(4):642-8.

46. Liu B, Fan Z, Edgerton SM et al. Metformin induces unique biological and molecular responses in triple negative breast cancer cells. Cell Cycle 2009 July 1;8(13):2031-40.

47. Hirsch HA, Iliopoulos D, Tsichlis PN, Struhl K. Metformin selectively targets cancer stem cells, and acts together with chemotherapy to block tumor growth and prolong remission. Cancer Res 2009 October 1;69(19):7507-11.

48. Liu J, Li M, Song B et al. Metformin inhibits renal cell carcinoma in vitro and in vivo xenograft. Urol Oncol 2013 February;31(2):264-70.

49. Kato K, Gong J, Iwama H et al. The antidiabetic drug Metformin inhibits gastric cancer cell proliferation in vitro and in vivo. Mol Cancer Ther 2012 March;11(3):549-60.

50. Qu Z, Zhang Y, Liao M, Chen Y, Zhao J, Pan Y. In vitro and in vivo antitumoral action of Metformin on hepatocellular carcinoma. Hepatol Res 2012 September;42(9):922-33.

51. Chaudhary SC, Kurundkar D, Elmets CA, Kopelovich L, Athar M. Metformin, an antidiabetic agent reduces growth of cutaneous squamous cell carcinoma by targeting mTOR signaling pathway. Photochem Photobiol 2012 September;88(5):1149-56.

52. Wu B, Li S, Sheng L et al. Metformin inhibits the development and metastasis of ovarian cancer. Oncol Rep 2012 September;28(3):903-8.

53. Kisfalvi K, Moro A, Sinnett-Smith J, Eibl G, Rozengurt E. Metformin inhibits the growth of human pancreatic cancer xenografts. Pancreas 2013 July;42(5):781-5.

54. Storozhuk Y, Hopmans SN, Sanli T et al. Metformin inhibits growth and enhances radiation response of non-small cell lung cancer (NSCLC) through ATM and AMPK. Br J Cancer 2013 May 28;108(10):2021-32.

55. Cufi S, Corominas-Faja B, Lopez-Bonet E et al. Dietary restriction-resistant human tumors harboring the PIK3CA-activating mutation H1047R are sensitive to Metformin. Oncotarget 2013 September;4(9):1484-95.

56. Zhang T, Guo P, Zhang Y et al. The antidiabetic drug Metformin inhibits the proliferation of bladder cancer cells in vitro and in vivo. Int J Mol Sci 2013;14(12):24603-18.

57. Nangia-Makker P, Yu Y, Vasudevan A et al. Metformin: a potential therapeutic agent for recurrent colon cancer. PLoS ONE 2014;9(1):e84369.

58. Miyoshi H, Kato K, Iwama H et al. Effect of the anti-diabetic drug Metformin in hepatocellular carcinoma in vitro and in vivo. Int J Oncol 2014 July;45(1):322-32.

59. Fujihara S, Kato K, Morishita A et al. Antidiabetic drug Metformin inhibits esophageal adenocarcinoma cell proliferation in vitro and in vivo. Int J Oncol 2015 May;46(5):2172-80.

60. Barbieri F, Thellung S, Ratto A et al. In vitro and in vivo antiproliferative activity of Metformin on stem-like cells isolated from spontaneous canine mammary carcinomas: translational implications for human tumors. BMC Cancer 2015;15:228.

61. Fujimori T, Kato K, Fujihara S et al. Antitumor effect of Metformin on cholangiocarcinoma: In vitro and in vivo studies. Oncol Rep 2015 December;34(6):2987-96.

62. Kato K, Iwama H, Yamashita T et al. The anti-diabetic drug Metformin inhibits pancreatic cancer cell proliferation in vitro and in vivo: Study of the microRNAs associated with the antitumor effect of Metformin. Oncol Rep 2016 March;35(3):1582-92.

63. Iliopoulos D, Hirsch HA, Struhl K. Metformin decreases the dose of chemotherapy for prolonging tumor remission in mouse xenografts involving multiple cancer cell types. Cancer Res 2011 May 1;71(9):3196-201.

64. Rocha GZ, Dias MM, Ropelle ER et al. Metformin amplifies chemotherapy-induced AMPK activation and antitumoral growth. Clin Cancer Res 2011 June 15;17(12):3993-4005.

65. Colquhoun AJ, Venier NA, Vandersluis AD et al. Metformin enhances the antiproliferative and apoptotic effect of bicalutamide in prostate cancer. Prostate Cancer Prostatic Dis 2012 December;15(4):346-52.

66. Lin CC, Yeh HH, Huang WL et al. Metformin enhances cisplatin cytotoxicity by suppressing signal transducer and activator of transcription-3 activity independently of the liver kinase B1-AMP-activated protein kinase pathway. Am J Respir Cell Mol Biol 2013 August;49(2):241-50.

67. Lin YC, Wu MH, Wei TT et al. Metformin sensitizes anticancer effect of dasatinib in head and neck squamous cell carcinoma cells through AMPK-dependent ER stress. Oncotarget 2014 January 15;5(1):298-308.

68. Ma J, Guo Y, Chen S et al. Metformin enhances tamoxifen-mediated tumor growth inhibition in ER-positive breast carcinoma. BMC Cancer 2014;14:172.

69. Honjo S, Ajani JA, Scott AW et al. Metformin sensitizes chemotherapy by targeting cancer stem cells and the mTOR pathway in esophageal cancer. Int J Oncol 2014 August;45(2):567-74.

70. Burke AR, Singh RN, Carroll DL et al. The resistance of breast cancer stem cells to conventional hyperthermia and their sensitivity to nanoparticle-mediated photothermal therapy. Biomaterials 2012 April;33(10):2961-70.

71. Hirsch HA, Iliopoulos D, Tsichlis PN, Struhl K. Metformin selectively targets cancer stem cells, and acts together with chemotherapy to block tumor growth and prolong remission. Cancer Res 2009 October 1;69(19):7507-11.

72. Bao B, Wang Z, Ali S et al. Metformin inhibits cell proliferation, migration and invasion by attenuating CSC function mediated by deregulating miRNAs in pancreatic cancer cells. Cancer Prev Res (Phila) 2012 March;5(3):355-64.

73. Chen G, Xu S, Renko K, Derwahl M. Metformin inhibits growth of thyroid carcinoma cells, suppresses self-renewal of derived cancer stem cells, and potentiates the effect of chemotherapeutic agents. J Clin Endocrinol Metab 2012 April;97(4):E510-E520.

74. Bednar F, Simeone DM. Metformin and cancer stem cells: old drug, new targets. Cancer Prev Res (Phila) 2012 March;5(3):351-4.

75. Song CW, Lee H, Dings RP et al. Metformin kills and radiosensitizes cancer cells and preferentially kills cancer stem cells. Sci Rep 2012;2:362.

76. Rattan R, Ali FR, Munkarah A. Metformin: an emerging new therapeutic option for targeting cancer stem cells and metastasis. J Oncol 2012;2012:928127.

77. Shank JJ, Yang K, Ghannam J et al. Metformin targets ovarian cancer stem cells in vitro and in vivo. Gynecol Oncol 2012 November;127(2):390-7.

78. Sato A, Sunayama J, Okada M et al. Glioma-initiating cell elimination by Metformin activation of FOXO3 via AMPK. Stem Cells Transl Med 2012 November;1(11):811-24.

79. Hirsch HA, Iliopoulos D, Struhl K. Metformin inhibits the inflammatory response associated with cellular transformation and cancer stem cell growth. Proc Natl Acad Sci U S A 2013 January 15;110(3):972-7.

80. Lonardo E, Cioffi M, Sancho P et al. Metformin targets the metabolic achilles heel of human pancreatic cancer stem cells. PLoS ONE 2013;8(10):e76518.

81. Zhang Y, Guan M, Zheng Z, Zhang Q, Gao F, Xue Y. Effects of Metformin on CD133+ colorectal cancer cells in diabetic patients. PLoS ONE 2013;8(11):e81264.

82. Zhu P, Davis M, Blackwelder AJ et al. Metformin selectively targets tumor-initiating cells in ErbB2-overexpressing breast cancer models. Cancer Prev Res (Phila) 2014 February;7(2):199-210.

83. Mohammed A, Janakiram NB, Brewer M et al. Antidiabetic Drug Metformin Prevents Progression of Pancreatic Cancer by Targeting in Part Cancer Stem Cells and mTOR Signaling. Transl Oncol 2013 December 1;6(6):649-59.

84. Lee H, Park HJ, Park CS et al. Response of breast cancer cells and cancer stem cells to Metformin and hyperthermia alone or combined. PLoS ONE 2014;9(2):e87979.

85. Najbauer J, Kraljik N, Nemeth P. Glioma stem cells: markers, hallmarks and therapeutic targeting by Metformin. Pathol Oncol Res 2014 October;20(4):789-97.

86. Bao B, Azmi AS, Ali S, Zaiem F, Sarkar FH. Metformin may function as anticancer agent via targeting cancer stem cells: the potential biological significance of tumor-associated miRNAs in breast and pancreatic cancers. Ann Transl Med 2014 June;2(6):59.

87. Barbieri F, Thellung S, Ratto A et al. In vitro and in vivo antiproliferative activity of Metformin on stem-like cells isolated from spontaneous canine mammary carcinomas: translational implications for human tumors. BMC Cancer 2015;15:228.

88. Chen X, Hu C, Zhang W et al. Metformin inhibits the proliferation, metastasis, and cancer stem-like sphere formation in osteosarcoma MG63 cells in vitro. Tumour Biol 2015 December;36(12):9873-83.

89. Mayer MJ, Klotz LH, Venkateswaran V. Metformin and prostate cancer stem cells: a novel therapeutic target. Prostate Cancer Prostatic Dis 2015 December;18(4):303-9.

90. Honjo S, Ajani JA, Scott AW et al. Metformin sensitizes chemotherapy by targeting cancer stem cells and the mTOR pathway in esophageal cancer. Int J Oncol 2014 August;45(2):567-74.

91. Chai X, Chu H, Yang X, Meng Y, Shi P, Gou S. Metformin Increases Sensitivity of Pancreatic Cancer Cells to Gemcitabine by Reducing CD133+ Cell Populations and Suppressing ERK/ P70S6K Signaling. Sci Rep 2015;5:14404.

92. McCarty MF, Contreras F. Increasing Superoxide Production and the Labile Iron Pool in Tumor Cells may Sensitize Them to Extracellular Ascorbate. Front Oncol 2014;4:249.

93. McCarty MF, Barroso-Aranda J, Contreras F. Practical strategies for suppressing hypoxia-inducible factor activity in cancer therapy. Med Hypotheses 2010 May;74(5):789-97.

94. Sinnberg T, Noor S, Venturelli S et al. The ROS-induced cytotoxicity of ascorbate is attenuated by hypoxia and HIF-1alpha in the NCI60 cancer cell lines. J Cell Mol Med 2014 March;18(3):530-41.

95. Hoffer LJ, Levine M, Assouline S et al. Phase I clinical trial of i.v. ascorbic acid in advanced malignancy. Ann Oncol 2008 November;19(11):1969-74.

96. Ma Y, Chapman J, Levine M, Polireddy K, Drisko J, Chen Q. High-dose parenteral ascorbate enhanced chemosensitivity of ovarian cancer and reduced toxicity of chemotherapy. Sci Transl Med 2014 February 5;6(222):222ra18.

97. Martin-Montalvo, A. Mercken, E.M., Mitchell, S.J. et al. (2013). Metformin improves healthspan and lifespan in mice. Nat Commun. 4:2192.

98. McCarty, M.F. (2004) Chronic activation of AMP-activated kinase as a strategy for slowing aging. Med Hypotheses. 63(2):334-9.

99. McCarty, M.F. (2014). AMPK activation--protean potential for boosting healthspan. Age (Dordr). April;36(2):641-63.

Caldwell B. Esselstyn, Jr. Delia Garcia Francisco Contreras Candice Kumai Michael Greger

HEALTHY LONG LIFE

DOCUMENTARY SERIES

"Daniel E. Kennedy's Healthy Long Life documentary series artfully shows the unfortunate consequences of transitioning from an agrarian, low cost, food-based health system of years past to an expensive high-tech health care system of time present. It is a unique inspiring documentary."

—T. Colin Campbell, PhD
Author, The China Study
Professor Emeritus, Cornell University

 tv

prime video

www.HealthyLongLife.com

"Healthy Long Life" App on
Apple TV Streaming Devices

HEALTHY LONG LIFE

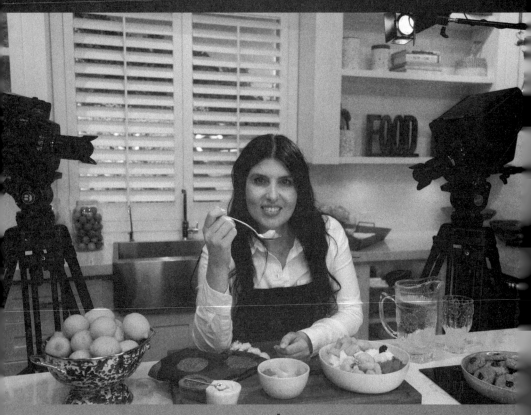

FREE RECIPE/COOKING APP
BY OASIS OF HOPE

Making healthy and delicious food has never been so easy.
Learn from Oasis of Hope's nutritionist, Rosa Contreras-Tessada,
and our teaching chef, on our free recipe app.
Search key words "Healthy Long Life" or use QR code.

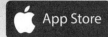
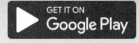

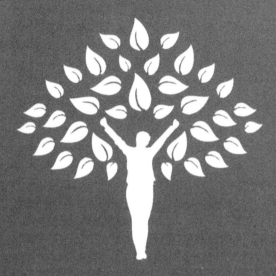

HEALTHY LONG LIFE

Watch Now on Prime Video

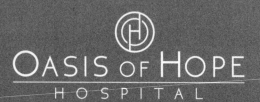

OASIS OF HOPE
HOSPITAL

For information about Oasis of Hope Hospital, our medical protocols, or to request a free treatment plan with an explanation of the therapies and costs, please contact our admissions department:

📞 1-888-500-HOPE (4673) USA

📞 01-800-02-OASIS (62747) México

📞 +1-619-690-8450 International

✉ contact@oasisofhope.com

🌐 www.oasisofhope.com

📘 @oasisofhopehospital

📷 @oasisofhopehospital

🐦 @hospitaloasis

▷ @oasisofhopehospital1963